Peripheral Neuropathy - Causes, Symptoms, and Treatment Options

Edited by Simona Maria Carmignano

Published in London, United Kingdom

Peripheral Neuropathy - Causes, Symptoms, and Treatment Options
http://dx.doi.org/10.5772/intechopen.1006229
Edited by Simona Maria Carmignano

Contributors
Andra-Elena Nica, Asma Hussain, Carmen Dobjanschi, Edith De Grand'Maison, Emilia Rusu, Gabriela Radulian, Hafsa Ahsan, Laura Collier, Mélanie Brassard, Oana Andreea Parliteanu, Patricia Bilodeau, Pauline Jardel, Robert Wright, Sahreen Anwar, Salim Zenkhri, Sivu Claudia, Sébastien S. Dufresne, Wajida Perveen

First published in London, United Kingdom, 2025 by IntechOpen
IntechOpen is the global imprint of INTECHOPEN LIMITED, registered in England and Wales, registration number: 11086078, 167-169 Great Portland Street, London, W1W 5PF, United Kingdom

For EU product safety concerns: IN TECH d.o.o., Prolaz Marije Krucifikse Kozulić 3, 51000 Rijeka, Croatia, info@intechopen.com or visit our website at intechopen.com.

British Library Cataloguing-in-Publication Data
A catalogue record for this book is available from the British Library

Peripheral Neuropathy - Causes, Symptoms, and Treatment Options
Edited by Simona Maria Carmignano
p. cm.
Print ISBN 978-1-83635-226-6
Online ISBN 978-1-83635-225-9
eBook (PDF) ISBN 978-1-83635-227-3

Meet the editor

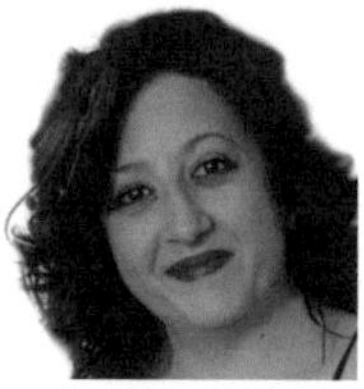

Dr. Simona Maria Carmignano is a specialist in Physical and Rehabilitation Medicine. She graduated with honors in Medicine and Surgery from the University of Chieti in 2012 and completed her specialization in 2017. She is a consultant physician at the CTR Therapeutic Rehabilitation Center in Tramutola and a contract professor at the University of Salerno. Her clinical and research interests focus on neurological rehabilitation, robotics in rehabilitation, and complex disorders of developmental age. Dr. Carmignano has authored multiple scientific articles and book chapters, contributing to the advancement of rehabilitation medicine.

Contents

Preface

Peripheral neuropathies are a heterogeneous group of disorders that significantly impact patients' quality of life, often manifesting as pain, sensory disturbances, or motor dysfunction. Their diagnosis and management require a nuanced understanding of anatomy, pathophysiology, and clinical reasoning—an intersection that this book aims to explore and clarify.

This volume brings together contributions from clinicians, surgeons, radiologists, and researchers, each offering unique perspectives grounded in both evidence and experience. The chapters address a range of topics—from the structural alterations of the ilioinguinal nerve in hernia patients, to the role of advanced imaging modalities in detecting nerve pathology, and the clinical evaluation and management of entrapment neuropathies such as carpal tunnel syndrome.

The content is organized into thematic sections designed to guide the reader through foundational knowledge, diagnostic challenges, and therapeutic strategies. We aim to provide a resource that is both scientifically rigorous and practically useful to a broad audience, including medical students, practicing clinicians, and specialists involved in the care of patients with peripheral nerve disorders.

We hope that this book will not only serve as a reference but will also stimulate further research and collaboration in the ongoing effort to improve outcomes for patients affected by peripheral neuropathies.

Simona Maria Carmignano
CTR Rehabilitation Therapy Center (Basilicata),
Adjunct Professor,
DIPMED,
University of Salerno,
Italy

Section 1

Entrapment Neuropathies

Chapter 1

Compression Neuropathy of the Ilioinguinal Nerves in Relation to Inguinal Hernia

Robert Wright and Laura Collier

Abstract

This chapter investigates the pathophysiology of ilioinguinal nerve and peripheral neuropathy in patients undergoing inguinal hernia repair. We hypothesize the abnormality of the ilioinguinal nerve in these patients with primary inguinal hernia. It inspects how nerve compression, most commonly resulting from the presence of an inguinal hernia compressing on the ilioinguinal nerve, leads to nerve damage and subsequent apparent enlargement. This chapter focuses on clinical implications from these changes, including the link between nerve enlargement and preoperative pain, as well as any potential long-term complications such as neuropathic discomfort or sensory changes. Through a detailed review of histological findings and surgical data from published articles, it aims to enhance understanding of all the mechanisms driving nerve-related pain in hernia repair patients.

Keywords: inguinal hernia, compression neuropathy, peripheral neuropathy, inguinal herniorrhaphy, ilioinguinal nerve enlargement, entrapment neuropathy

1. Introduction

The initial source of preoperative pain in inguinal hernia repair patients remains a significant clinical mystery. Despite being common among hernia repair patients, the underlying cause behind the pain associated with hernias is unknown. Historically surgeons have been taught that the nerves affected by inguinal hernias, primarily the ilioinguinal nerve, appear normal upon examination. The pain is summed up to be from mechanical compression or irritation of muscle, ligament, or bone. However, this traditional notion lacks vital histological evidence in terms of explaining the origin of this preoperative pain. Previously, it was presumed that these nerves remained structurally intact and functional, but recent conclusions from my research challenges this idea.

The hypothesis we are testing is that a significant portion of the preoperative pain that inguinal hernia patients report stems from pressure on the ilioinguinal nerve. This could also potentially impact the genitofemoral and iliohypogastric nerves, all of which also traverse the inguinal region. Nerve enlargement at the external inguinal ring in primary inguinal hernia was initially defined as presenting in 34% of patients, most commonly occurring with the ilioinguinal nerve at the external inguinal ring [1]. These nerves are sensory and could result in the pain experienced, although very little histological data has been provided to confirm any structural changes or damage. Until recently, it was assumed that these nerves, although compressed, were otherwise "normal" during surgical inspections. This belief persisted without in-depth analysis, relying instead on clinical observations that suggested only irritation to the nerves rather than damage to the structure of the nerve. However, there has been new compelling evidence found through histological findings that these nerves in some patients are often not normal as previously depicted. This evidence proves to be consistent with Sunderland grade three neuropathy. This type of neuropathy is significant because it is a type of permanent nerve damage and can result in chronic pain in a sensory nerve such as the ilioinguinal nerve. The surgeon is many times blamed for the postoperative pain. The surgeon is also instructed to leave these "normal" nerves intact during surgery, but what if they are in fact permanently damaged preoperatively?

2. Summary of available literature

2.1 First nerve resection

While performing an open inguinal hernia repair many years ago, one of us (RW) observed an ilioinguinal nerve that was tightly tethered to the external inguinal ring and the spermatic cord with substantial enlargement of the nerve. This patient had been experiencing considerable preoperative pain. Despite recommendations from the Hernia Society to leave the nerves alone, Robert Wright believed that resecting the nerve was necessary to reduce the potential of chronic pain from a chronically damaged nerve. This was the first time the surgeon (RW) had resected a nerve during a hernia repair. It had been emphasized from prior training that these nerves were considered normal and were to be pushed aside to allow repair and then returned to their original positions once the hernia was removed. Recent findings have now demonstrated that this approach of pushing aside the nerves may contribute to higher incidence of chronic pain, likely due to nerve stretch, and interruption of blood supply to the nerve [2].

The patient's nerve was sent for histological examination where the pathologist labeled it as a "traumatic neuroma." A traumatic neuroma results from transection of a nerve, and this resulting neuroma indicated that this nerve was severely damaged by the external ring and forces related to the inguinal hernia. In following years further ilioinguinal nerve resection occurred more routinely, particularly when nerve enlargement was evident at the external inguinal ring, even if fibrosis was not severe.

2.2 Ilioinguinal nerve enlargement at the external ring is common in primary inguinal hernia

The first publication regarding this phenomenon is titled "Inguinal Neuritis is Common in Primary Inguinal Hernia" [1]. This article is an evaluation retrospectively of 100 consecutive open inguinal hernia repairs. It was found that 34% of these patients exhibited an enlarged ilioinguinal nerve that was resected. Enlargement occurred in the ilioinguinal nerve in 88% of the patients in this study and of those patients with enlarged nerves 83% were enlarged distal to the external inguinal ring. One percent of these patients had two nerves showing enlargement. Histologically, myxoid was present on H&E staining, which demonstrated edema. The pathologist also identified perineural fibrosis and thickening of the perineurium. No inflammation, neoplasia, or incidences of Raynaud bodies were found. This proposed nerve damage was occurring in 34% of the patients. After 35 nerve resections, the pathologist labeled only one of the nerves as "normal," which comes solely from H&E stains done by community pathologists.

This study provided circumstantial evidence of the pathological process happening to these nerves and indicated that they are in fact not normal. At this time there was not a term for this; however, the editor of Hernia wanted it to be referred to as "inguinal neuritis" even though there were no inflammatory cells found in the histology.

These findings were followed up, subsequentially in a retrospective study of 30 patients with recurrent inguinal hernias repaired in an open fashion. These findings were directly compared with the prior study of 100 patients. In the recurrent hernias, enlargement of a nerve was found in 66% of patients versus 34% in the original paper; 69% of these patients showed enlargement in the ilioinguinal nerve versus 88% in the non-recurrent patients. In 70% of patients this enlargement occurred at the external ring favorably comparing with 83% in the primary hernia. Two nerves were involved in 20% of patients versus 1% in the nonrecurrent patients. Thus, the enlargement of the nerves was more common in recurrent hernias, and showed a very similar distribution, and was more likely to occur in more than one nerve.

These two studies provide circumstantial evidence of the proximity of the ilioinguinal nerve interacting, with the external inguinal ring. This evidence seems to be associated with nerve enlargement, as is commonly seen in compression neuropathy, and histological findings also are suggestive of nerve damage.

Compressive neuropathy has been extensively studied in human subjects and in animals, both experimentally and in autopsy studies [3–12]. The phenomenon of compressive neuropathy occurs in areas where pressure is exerted upon the nerve, usually by a ligament or tendon in a confined space. When this nerve is compressed, its microvasculature within the endoneurium is substantially diminished as it relies mostly on diffusion rather than blood vessels. The compression impedes or reverses flow of nutrients from the epineurium or perineurium, therefore, allowing ischemic injury to the nerve within the compressed segment. Grossly, this is usually associated with a smaller diameter of the nerve within the compressed segment and distal enlargement of the nerve grossly. Histologically this can be associated with perineural fibrosis, endoneurial edema depicted as myxoid. In carpal tunnel, there are typically development of Raynaud bodies. The histological evaluation of the inguinal canal has now begun and is summarized in this publication.

2.3 Pain and compression neuropathy in primary inguinal hernia

These papers were followed up with a prospective evaluation of 35 inguinal hernia patients who had preoperative pain evaluated with a validated hernia pain score, the Carolina's Comfort Scale [13]. This study was done with H&E staining again, evaluating the nerve just proximal to the external ring versus the nerve distal to the external inguinal ring if that nerve demonstrated enlargement distally. This study was with primary hernias, and we found that 63% of the patients had a distally enlarged nerve just beyond the external inguinal ring. Diameter of the nerve was measured histologically and correlated with pain scores on the Carolina's Comfort Scale.

In this study the results showed when the nerve grossly appeared enlarged at the external ring there was a measurable increase in nerve specific diameter and overall diameter compared with the proximal nerve. So, the distal nerve's specific diameter significantly increased $P < 0.005$, and the distal overall diameter is also significantly increased just beyond the external ring $P < 0.001$. When the nerve was increased in size, there was a correlation of pain with the increased diameter of nerve with 4/8 Carolina's Comfort Scale pain scores being elevated [13]. Pain sitting up $P < 0.003$, pain walking $P < 0.002$, pain with daily activities $P < 0.04$, and pain with walking upstairs $P < 0.05$.

Overall diameter of the distal nerve (which is evident to the surgeon grossly as nerve enlargement during the surgery) is correlated with preoperative pain, namely pain laying down $P < 0.01$, pain sitting up $P < 0.03$, pain with daily activities of living $P < 0.02$, and pain walking $P < 0.007$. Thus, preoperative pain scores correlate in 4/8 activity categories when the surgeon can visually detect gross enlargement of the ilioinguinal nerve at the external ring during open repair. None of the typical pains commonly associated with hernia onset (pain exercising, pain when coughing, and pain when bending over) correlate with increased nerve diameter or increased overall diameter. This indicates that these early pains are not associated with nerve enlargement. Thus, the grossly enlarged nerve at the external inguinal ring can predictably be associated with higher levels of preoperative pain, particularly with low levels of activity.

This study also showed that there is a negative correlation with nerve specific diameter and increasing ages associated with lower pain scores when nerve specific diameter is considered $P < 0.001$.

2.4 Groin anatomy, preoperative pain, and compression neuropathy in primary inguinal hernia: What really matters

Further investigation of this phenomenon led to anatomical evaluation of patients with their preoperative pain. This was a prospective study of 143 consecutive primary inguinal hernia patients, whose Carolina's Comfort scores had been recorded. Detailed anatomical analysis of the hernia was also described and recorded at the time of repair. These factors were evaluated in a prospective larger series to see what anatomical factors are associated with nerve enlargement and pain. Patients with enlarged nerves were then compared to patients with non-enlarged nerves for statistical evaluation. The hernia anatomy was then evaluated using the European Hernia Society classification, which documents hernia size (no hernia detected, <1.5 cm, <3 cm, >3 cm) and hernia type (direct or indirect). Other evaluations were also made to indicate the hernia incarceration status. This included the degree of fibrosis of the external oblique fascia at the external ring, method of hernia determination, status of genital branch nerve, ilioinguinal nerve trajectory, and iliohypogastric nerve course. The data was then evaluated by a statistician to determine any statistical significance between the intraoperative anatomical information and the preoperative pain and patient classification information [14]. Anatomical variations were examined as well as preoperative pain levels between patients with enlarged and non-enlarged nerves. The means of groups were compared using independent samples t-tests for independent measures utilizing robust sandwich variance estimator to account for multiple observations per patient. The P values were then calculated using the Bonferroni adjustment method due to the high number of dependent variables examined. This reduces the likelihood of type 1 statistical error in the results. Confidence intervals were also calculated to increase our confidence that any difference or lack thereof between groups is true and not due to random variance [14].

In this study, 63% of patients exhibited enlarged nerves at the external inguinal ring. Fibrosis of the external inguinal ring involving the ilioinguinal nerve was the single anatomical factor relating to predictable increased diameter size of the nerve at the external inguinal ring $P < 0.001$. Eighty-one percent of the patients were found to have histological abnormalities if the nerve grossly was enlarged. Those were mostly perineural fibrosis and endoneurial fibrosis on H&E stain. In terms of pain, enlargement of the nerve at the external ring was correlated with pain "most of the time" $P < 0.0017$ versus nerves that were not enlarged. This exhaustive study clearly demonstrated that fascia interaction with the nerve seems to be the most important anatomical determinant of nerve enlargement, and nerve enlargement is most positively correlated with higher preoperative pain scores.

2.5 Why do inguinal hernia patients have pain? Histology points to compression neuropathy

In follow-up of this study, another prospective study was carried out with 35 patients undergoing inguinal hernia repair. This was an H&E stain study for myeloid as a surrogate for edema indicating injury of the nerve versus Carolina's Comfort Scale pain scores. Again, of the 35 patients 22 demonstrated thickened nerve segment at the external ring (63% of the total). They also had increased pain scores, which were correlated positively with increased nerve diameter, increased myxoid in the perineurium, increased myoid in the endoneurium, and increased fascicle counts. The myxoid in the perineurium and endoneurium was more pronounced than in the epineurium. The epineurium has arterial and venous blood supply, whereas the perineurium and endoneurium rely on diffusion of nutrients. Without the benefit of arterial and venous blood supply and the location and diameter of evidence of edema point to compressive neuropathy as the underlying physiology affecting the nerve.

Other studies have demonstrated that the preoperative pain experienced by patients undergoing inguinal hernia repair may function as a significant predictor of postoperative pain [2, 15, 16]. This is specifically prevalent when discussing the underlying nerve damage revealed by recent histological findings. A new growing body of evidence proposes that primary inguinal hernia causes pressure-induced peripheral nerve injury. The new histological examinations of primary hernia in an autopsy series display deterioration in unnamed tissue nerves including fibrosis, thickening of the perineurium sheath, and fatty dystrophy of axons [17, 19].

If preoperative pain is motivated by irreversible nerve damage, such as Sutherland-Sunderland grade 3 neuropathy, the severity of damage to the ilioinguinal nerve and other associated nerves may predispose patients to chronic postoperative pain or discomfort. This link between preoperative pain and postoperative pain potentially could result from altered sensory pathways that could amplify pain perception after the hernia has been removed [18–20].

2.6 Reduced fascicle area demonstrated in ilioinguinal nerves resected from primary inguinal herniorrhaphy patients as evidence of compression neuropathy

With this evidence as background, we finally got some funding for special staining of the nerves. The next study involved prospective analysis of 30 consecutive primary inguinal hernia patients. Staining of the ilioinguinal nerve was done at three locations: proximal to the inguinal canal, in the inguinal canal, and just distal to the inguinal canal at the external inguinal ring. Masson's trichrome stain was utilized to look for evidence of collagen deposition and further evaluate cross sectional areas of the nerves. This study demonstrated that the fascicles cross-sectional area within the canal segment is significantly smaller than the proximal segment which is unaffected by the trajectory of the hernia and its pressure ($P < 0.016$). The collagen content seemed to be similar throughout the nerve. However, from this study, we concluded that the apparent enlargement of the segment of the ilioinguinal nerve just distal to the external ring was an apparent enlargement. This segment was actually similar in diameter to the proximal nerve and that in fact the canal segment nerve was smaller, likely due to the compression. This is typically seen as mentioned above in compressive neuropathy where there is a smaller nerve diameter where the compression occurs and apparent distal enlargement of the nerve. Collagen deposition is uniformly distributed, so the size difference in the canal segment fascicle may be due to axon loss which is common in compression neuropathy (**Table 1**) [23].

Sample location	*N*[*]	Proximal (control)	Canal	Distal	Canal vs. proximal	Canal vs. distal	Proximal vs. distal
		Mean (mm^2)	Mean (mm^2)	Mean (mm^2)	P	P	P
Total nerve cross-sectional area	23	0.130	0.170	0.138	0.109	0.190	0.655
Total fascicle cross-sectional area	24	3.426	2.482	3.121	**0.016**	0.107	0.350
Total collagen cross-sectional area	24	0.162	0.162	0.162	1	1	1

[*]*N is calculated with outliers removed; Numbers in bold indicate significance.*

Table 1.
Measurements of the total nerve cross-sectional area, total fascicle cross-sectional area, and total collagen cross-sectional area at the three sample sites.

2.7 Axon loss and collagen deposition in the ilioinguinal nerve resected from primary inguinal herniorrhaphy patients

Another study focused on the axon loss and collagen deposition in the ilioinguinal nerve resected from primary inguinal herniorrhaphy patients. Prior to this study ilioinguinal nerve enlargement at the external ring had not been examined for axon loss in conjunction with neural collagen. The purpose of this research was to find evidence of compression neuropathy in the ilioinguinal nerve associated with primary inguinal hernias. This study observed 10 male patients with primary inguinal hernias that displayed gross nerve enlargement during inguinal herniorrhaphies. Samples of the ilioinguinal nerve were resected to include the proximal (control), canal, and distal segments with respect to the external ring. These nerve samples were then stained to detect changes in axon appearance and collagen content.

The results indicated by the tables below display moderate to severe axon loss in 50% and 80% of patients, respectively in the canal and distal segments extracted. The canal segment conveys increased collagen content when compared to the control ($P < 0.02$). The canal and distal segments also had increases in fascicular areas compared to the control ($P < 0.0058$, $P < 0.0098$) (**Figure 1** and **Tables 2** and **3**).

The data found from this study explained how the exposure of the nerve in the canal segment to primary inguinal hernias is associated with moderate to severe axon loss. It also had increased fascicular areas attributed to collagen deposition (i.e., fibrosis). This process is consistent with compression neuropathy, which supports the hypothesis that these nerves are not normal in patients with visible nerve enlargement.

Histological examination of these nerves has revealed a marked reduction in fascicle size, along with signs of fibrosis, myxoid changes, and nerve fiber degeneration. These are all indicative of nerve damage caused by sustained compression. These structural changes suggest that the visibly enlarged ilioinguinal nerve, which often is correlated in hernia-related pain, may suffer from compression neuropathy prior to surgical intervention. This compression can lead to axonal damage, resulting in neuropathy that manifests as persistent pain and sensory dysfunction. This is consistent with compression neuropathy, which is associated with preoperative pain with a certain segment of patients also developing chronic pain. The identification of these changes in nerve structure provides insight into the underlying mechanisms of preoperative pain and highlights the need for careful nerve assessment during hernia repair.

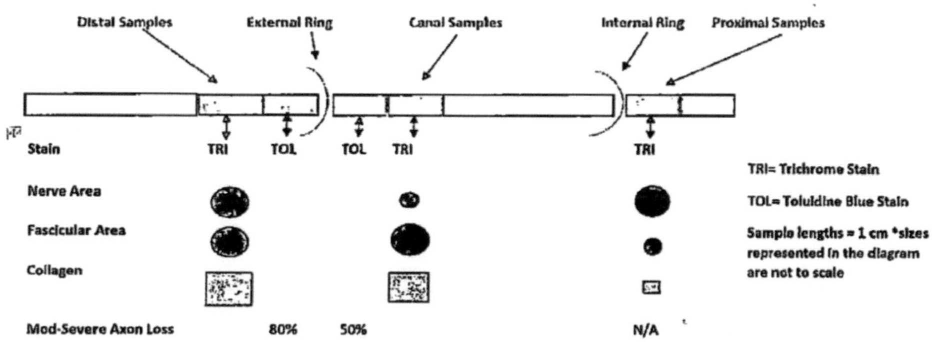

Figure 1.
The figure above depicts a graphical abstract displaying the collagen content, areas, and axon loss of the ilioinguinal nerve through the ilioinguinal canal. The location along the nerve displays the impact it has on these variables based on different types of stains done to test axon loss and collagen deposition.

Measurement	Nerve segment	Mean	+/-
Total nerve area (mm^2)	Proximal	3.32	1.48
	Canal	1.99	1.03
	Distal	2.61	0.087
Total fascicular area (mm^2)	Proximal	0.129	0.062
	Canal	0.198	0.109
	Distal	0.177	0.087
Total collagen area (mm^2)	Proximal	0.563	0.142
	Canal	0.605	0.071
	Distal	0.599	0.072

Table 2.
Nerve areas and collagen content from trichrome stain by nerve segment.

Measurement	Segments compared	P-Value
Total nerve area (mm^2)	Canal < distal	P < 0.04*
	Canal < proximal	P < 0.006*
Total fascicular area (mm^2)	Canal > proximal	P < 0.0058*
	Distal > proximal	P < 0.0098*
Total collagen area (mm^2)	Canal > proximal	P < 0.02*
	Distal > proximal	P < 0.18

**indicates statistical significance.*

Table 3.
Trichrome stain findings from measured areas and collagen content by nerve segment.

Despite the understanding from most surgeons that preoperative pain is primarily due to mechanical compression or irritation, recent histological findings now suggest that the nerves involved particularly the enlarged ilioinguinal nerve suffer from structural damage. This damage includes fibrosis, nerve enlargement, and axonal degeneration similar to Sutherland-Sunderland grade three neuropathy. These findings challenged the previous notion that these nerves appear to be "normal" during surgery.

A key factor in understanding the compression occurring on these nerves is comprehending the nerve anatomy of the nerves affected and the rationale behind sampling specific segments. Inguinal hernia repair typically involves the iliohypogastric, ilioinguinal, and genitofemoral nerves, which all traverse the inguinal region and can be subject to compression or damage. The iliohypogastric nerve provides sensory and motor innervation to the abdominal muscles and groin. The ilioinguinal nerve supplies sensation to the groin and inner thigh. These nerves are typically in close proximity to the inguinal hernia and are susceptible to injury. The genitofemoral nerve supplies sensation to the skin of the anterior scrotal area in males, mons pubis in women, and the upper segment of the anterior thigh in both males and females. This nerve may also be impacted by the hernia. When discussing compression neuropathy of these nerves specific segments of the nerves are targeted in order to assess structural damage caused by the compression. The segment of nerve that is chosen to be sampled is typically based on the area's most commonly affected by hernia-related compression. This typically means focusing on the nerve segments near the external inguinal ring where the pressure from the hernia and surrounding tissues is most prominent. By analyzing these specific areas of nerve segment, surgeons can better understand the extent of damage to the nerves and its connection to preoperative and postoperative pain.

3. Conclusions

We feel that the above studies demonstrate compressive neuropathy. This is evident with perineural fibrosis on H&E stain, myxoid in the perineurium and endoneurium on H&E stain with discrepancy in nerve diameters. The larger distal nerve diameters are correlated with higher pain scores. Pain and sensory changes are characterized of compressive neuropathy. Additionally, with evidence of axon loss of 50% and 80% involving the ilioinguinal nerve when the ilioinguinal nerve is enlarged at the external ring, this is direct evidence of Sunderland class III nerve damage. This is irreversible nerve damage and frequently is associated with chronic sensory changes including pain. If the surgeon's goal in relation to primary inguinal hernia is to reduce the potential for chronic postoperative pain, then the intervention possibly needed is early surgery before compression neuropathy is allowed to occur as such, and the concept of watching and waiting is called into question [24–25].

These series of papers have demonstrated that in primary inguinal hernia, when a surgeon is able to discern visible enlargement of the ilioinguinal nerve at the external inguinal ring, they are likely looking at patients who have higher preoperative pain scores. Those patients also have axon loss, perineural fibrosis, and edema within the nerve. These patients are likely to already have experienced Sunderland class III nerve injury from the hernia itself, and it is my practice to routinely resect these nerves in hopes of preventing postoperative pain rather than leaving these nerves intact. The American Hernia Society has one of its major goals to prevent postoperative pain in hernia patients, and they have embraced pragmatic selective nerve removal during open inguinal hernia repair leaving it up to the surgeon's judgment [26]. These histologic and pain and anatomic findings all should be taken into consideration by the surgeon at the time of primary inguinal hernia repair in assessing whether pragmatic removal is necessary or not.

Since none of the typical pains associated with hernia onset (pain exercising, pain when coughing, and pain when bending over) correlate with increased nerve diameter and compression neuropathy, this would be the appropriate time to operate. Pain at rest may mean irreparable damage.

This chapter does not address postoperative pain, but there are many factors that can contribute to it. One of these factors occurs in as many as 63% of patients and may relate to preoperative compressive neuropathy but other surgical factors can also play a role including mobilization of the nerve, nerve placement after repair, nerve contact with the mesh used, and suture or tack contact with the nerve. This is why postoperative pain is difficult to nail down to one thing in terms of its etiology. The key to understanding post-herniorrhaphy pain in the groin may be related to compression neuropathy existing prior to hernia repair.

The studies completed in these articles did not have a large funding and are limited by certain factors. This implies that these studies need to be repeated in multiple hospitals, with outstanding stains, particularly with the toluidine blue stain since it will help get a better depiction on axon loss. Another piece of information that should be taken into account is age as it has been suggested that it has correlations with nerve status. There also needs to be further studies comparing male vs. female since all the studies in these papers solely looked at males. Finally postoperative pain evaluation in patients with operative removal of nerves showing evidence of compression neuropathy who undergo neurectomy, instead nerve retention must be done to determine best course of action.

The histologic findings described above do strengthen the notion of a triple neurectomy being a useful adjunct in solving post-herniorrhaphy pain. It would be instructive if this type of nerve analysis was done on patients who underwent triple neurectomy for post-herniorrhaphy pain to see if these changes are present, certainly if present the question would be whether they developed as a result of the operation or whether they were preexisting. Since all of those patients are experiencing pain, the question is whether that is neurologic pain or somatic pain or related to the mesh itself and a histologic evaluation of those nerves particularly looking for axon loss, myxoid presence, and fibrosis might help answer that question.

Prior studies regarding neurectomy during inguinal hernia repairs have shown mixed results recording a decrease in pain. To my knowledge none of them show an increase in pain unless all three nerves are removed. It may be that removal of normal nerves does not render any improvement, and since a lot of patients have normal nerves, it would take a very larger study to demonstrate improvement with neurectomy, but if neurectomy were done selectively on patients who were likely to have compressive neuropathy there may be an advantage in a select group of hernia patients. That number may be as high as 60%, according to these studies.

Currently the choice of whether a hernia is repaired laparoscopically, robotically, or open is largely left up between the patient and the surgeon's comfort level, experience, and clinical judgment. If prospective studies demonstrate that postoperative long-term herniorrhaphy pain can be diminished by selective neurectomy in patients who are likely to have compressive neuropathy, there may be a role for patients with higher preoperative pain scores to choose an open route so that those nerves could be evaluated directly and resected at the time of surgery.

Overall, these studies regarding the ilioinguinal nerve will help future clinicians to understand that these nerves may not be normal, and hopefully this will give a better understanding to surgeons about what they are seeing during open surgery. This may also give researchers more paths to evaluate compression neuropathy and also further help long-term studies to inspect the outcomes of pragmatic removal of these nerves.

Author details

Robert Wright[1] and Laura Collier[2]

1 Cascade Hernia Institute, Puyallup, WA, USA

2 University of Oregon, Portland, OR, USA

*Address all correspondence to: bob@meridiansurgerycenterwa.com

References

[1] Wright RC, Sanders E. Inguinal neuritis is common in primary inguinal hernia. Hernia. 2011;**15**(4):393-398. DOI: 10.1007/s10029-011-0807-z. Epub 2011 Mar 27

[2] Reinpold WM, Nehls J, Eggert A. Nerve management and chronic pain after open inguinal hernia repair: A prospective two phase study. Annals of Surgery. 2011;**254**(1):163-168. DOI: 10.1097/SLA.0b013e31821d4a2d

[3] Nakamichi KI, Tachibana S. Enlarged median nerve in idiopathic carpal tunnel syndrome. Muscle & Nerve. 2000;**23**(11):1713-1718. DOI: 10.1002/1097-4598(200011)23:11<1713::aid-mus7>3.0.co;2-g

[4] Shapiro BE, Preston DC. Entrapment and compressive neuropathies. The Medical Clinics of North America. 2009;**93**(2):285-315, vii. DOI: 10.1016/j.mcna.2008.09.009

[5] Arnold WD, Elsheikh BH. Entrapment neuropathies. Neurologic Clinics. 2013;**31**(2):405-424. DOI: 10.1016/j.ncl.2013.01.002. Epub 2013 Feb 8

[6] Rempel D, Dahlin L, Lundborg G. Pathophysiology of nerve compression syndromes: Response of peripheral nerves to loading. The Journal of Bone and Joint Surgery. American Volume. 1999;**81**(11):1600-1610. DOI: 10.2106/00004623-199911000-00013

[7] Mackinnon SE, Dellon AL, Hudson AR, Hunter DA. Chronic human nerve compression—A histological assessment. Neuropathology and Applied Neurobiology. 1986;**12**(6):547-565. DOI: 10.1111/j.1365-2990.1986.tb00159.x

[8] Neary D, Eames RA. The pathology of ulnar nerve compression in man. Neuropathology and Applied Neurobiology. 1975;**116**(1):23 32. DOI: 10.1111/j.1365-2990.1975.tb00379.x

[9] Rempel DM, Diao E. Entrapment neuropathies: Pathophysiology and pathogenesis. Journal of Electromyography and Kinesiology. 2004;**14**(1):71-75. DOI: 10.1016/j.jelekin.2003.09.009

[10] Mackinnon SE. Pathophysiology of nerve compression. Hand Clinics. 2002;**18**(2):231-241. DOI: 10.1016/s0749-0712(01)00012-9

[11] Thatte MR, Mansukhani KA. Compressive neuropathy in the upper limb. Indian Journal of Plastic Surgery. 2011;**44**(2):283-297. DOI: 10.4103/0970-0358.85350

[12] Lundborg G, Myers R, Powell H. Nerve compression injury and increased endoneurial fluid pressure: A "miniature compartment syndrome". Journal of Neurology, Neurosurgery, and Psychiatry. 1983;**46**(12):1119-1124. DOI: 10.1136/jnnp.46.12.1119

[13] Heniford BT, Lincourt AE, Walters AL, Colavita PD, Belyansky I, Kercher KW, et al. Carolinas comfort scale as a measure of hernia repair quality of life: A reappraisal utilizing 3788 international patients. Annals of Surgery. 2018;**267**(1):171-176. DOI: 10.1097/SLA.0000000000002027

[14] Wright R, Salisbury T, Landes J. Groin anatomy, preoperative pain, and compression neuropathy in primary inguinal hernia: What really matters. American Journal of Surgery. 2019;**217**(5):873-877. DOI: 10.1016/j.amjsurg.2019.02.017. Epub 2019 Feb 27

[15] Aasvang E, Kehlet H. Chronic postoperative pain: The case of inguinal herniorrhaphy. British Journal of Anaesthesia. 2005;**95**(1):69-76. DOI: 10.1093/bja/aei019. Epub 2004 Nov 5

[16] O'Dwyer PJ, Alani A, McConnachie A. Groin hernia repair: Postherniorrhaphy pain. World Journal of Surgery. 2005;**29**(8):1062-1065. DOI: 10.1007/s00268-005-7903-0

[17] Neary D, Ochoa J, Gilliatt RW. Sub-clinical entrapment neuropathy in man. Journal of the Neurological Sciences. 1975;**24**(3):283-298. DOI: 10.1016/0022-510x(75)90248-8

[18] Wright R, Born DE, D'Souza N, Hurd L, Gill R. Daniel Wright, why do inguinal hernia patients have pain? Histology points to compression neuropathy. The American Journal of Surgery. 2017;**213**(5):975-982. ISSN:0002-9610. DOI: 10.1016/j.amjsurg.2017.03.013

[19] Wright R, Born DE, D'Souza N, Hurd L, Gill R, Wright D. Pain and compression neuropathy in primary inguinal hernia. Hernia. 2017;**21**(5):715-722. DOI: 10.1007/s10029-017-1641-8. Epub 2017 Aug 17

[20] Axon Loss and Collagen Deposition in the Ilioinguinal Nerve Resected from Primary Inguinal Herniorrhaphy Patients

[21] Sunderland S. The intraneural topography of the radial, median and ulnar nerves. Brain. 1945;**68**:243-299. DOI: 10.1093/brain/68.4.243

[22] Jabaley ME, Wallace WH, Heckler FR. Internal topography of major nerves of the forearm and hand: A current view. The Journal of Hand Surgery. 1980;**5**(1):1-18. DOI: 10.1016/s0363-5023(80)80035-9

[23] Wright R, Born DE, Sanders T, Landes J, Salisbury T, Kumar AS, et al. Reduced fascicle area demonstrated in ilioinguinal nerves resected from primary inguinal herniorrhaphy patients as evidence of compression neuropathy. Pain Research & Management. 2024;**2024**:3339753. DOI: 10.1155/2024/3339753

[24] Chung L, Norrie J, O'Dwyer PJ. Long-term follow-up of patients with a painless inguinal hernia from a randomized clinical trial. The British Journal of Surgery. 2011;**98**(4):596-599. DOI: 10.1002/bjs.7355. Epub 2010 Nov 30

[25] Fitzgibbons RJ Jr, Ramanan B, Arya S, Turner SA, Li X, Gibbs JO, et al. Long-term results of a randomized controlled trial of a nonoperative strategy (watchful waiting) for men with minimally symptomatic inguinal hernias. Annals of Surgery. 2013;**258**(3):508-515. DOI: 10.1097/SLA.0b013e3182a19725

[26] Alferi S, Amid PK, Campanelli G, et al. International guidelines for prevention and management of post-operative chronic pain following inguinal hernia surgery. Hernia. 2011;**15**(3):239 249. DOI: 10.1007/s10029-011-0798-9

Section 2

Diagnostic and Interventional Approaches

Chapter 2

Radiologic Perspectives in Peripheral Neuropathy: Imaging Modality, Diagnostic, and Interventional Insights

Salim Zenkhri

Abstract

Peripheral neuropathy is a debilitating disorder of the peripheral nervous system, requiring a multidisciplinary approach to accurately characterize nerve disease and guide management. Radiology has revolutionized this field, offering unparalleled insights into nerve pathology. The etiology of peripheral neuropathy spans metabolic disorders, autoimmune conditions, infections, neurotoxic exposures, and traumatic or compression injuries, each presenting distinct challenges. Patients often endure pain, paresthesia, numbness, and motor dysfunction, underscoring the urgency of precise diagnosis and targeted treatment before irreversible nerve damage. Advanced imaging techniques, such as high-resolution ultrasound and magnetic resonance neurography, provide exceptional clarity in visualizing nerve architecture, enabling early detection of entrapments, nerve injury, or infiltrative processes. Advanced imaging modalities, including diffusion tensor imaging, facilitate the detection of microstructural nerve damage. Beyond its diagnostic role, radiology enhances accuracy in image-guided interventions, such as nerve biopsies, targeted injections, and radiofrequency or cryoablation. When integrated with clinical and electrophysiological data, radiologic insights support personalized treatment strategies. This chapter underscores the semiology and the role of nerve imaging as a cornerstone in diagnosing and managing complex peripheral neuropathy, combining precision diagnostics with impactful interventions to improve patient outcomes.

Keywords: peripheral nerve disease, ultrasound, magnetic resonance imaging, neurography, diffusion magnetic resonance, diffusion tensor imaging

1. Introduction

Peripheral neuropathy (PNP) is a prevalent and complex condition with diverse etiologies, including metabolic disorders, autoimmune diseases, infections, neurotoxic exposures, hereditary conditions, neoplasia, and trauma-related nerve injuries [1]. It affects over 8% of the general population, with prevalence increasing to 15% in individuals over 40 years of age. Among its subtypes, distal symmetric polyneuropathies are the most common, frequently arising as long-term complications of systemic diseases, particularly diabetic neuropathy [2]. Notably, up to 46% of cases are idiopathic, underscoring the diagnostic challenges associated with PNP [3].

A systematic approach is essential for diagnosing PNP, integrating clinical history, physical examination, laboratory investigations, and electrodiagnostic studies [4, 5]. Laboratory tests help identify metabolic, autoimmune, infectious, or toxic causes [5]. Electrophysiologic studies further distinguish neuropathies based on chronicity, focality, and axonal versus demyelinating involvement. However, they have key limitations, such as imprecise lesion localization, restricted assessment of lesion extent, and inadequate evaluation of spatial distribution, all crucial for accurate diagnosis [6]. Moreover, electrophysiology cannot reliably differentiate between distal nerve lesions affecting the entire nerve cross-section and proximal lesions selectively involving specific fascicles. This limitation arises from the internal somatotopic organization of peripheral nerves, which mirrors the spatial arrangement of motor and sensory tracts in the central nervous system [7].

Advanced imaging techniques, particularly ultrasound (US) and magnetic resonance neurography (MRN), have transformed the evaluation of PNP by enabling direct visualization of peripheral nerves. These non-invasive modalities help overcome the limitations of traditional electrodiagnostic tests by providing structural and microstructural insights into nerve pathology [8]. Furthermore, radiology plays an expanding role in therapeutic interventions, including image-guided nerve blocks, targeted injections, and precise biopsy guidance, enhancing both diagnostic accuracy and treatment strategies [9, 10].

Given the heterogeneity of PNP, its diagnostic challenges require a multidisciplinary approach [5]. This review provides an overview of peripheral nerve imaging, beginning with an exploration of key imaging modalities and emerging technologies. It then highlights their clinical applications, emphasizing their role in enhancing diagnostic precision and guiding targeted management strategies.

2. Basic imaging anatomy and approach to peripheral nerve assessment

Peripheral nerves consist of bundles of nerve fibers that relay signals between the central nervous system and the body. They are organized into three connective tissue layers: the epineurium, which forms the dense external sheath that provides structural support; the perineurium, a dense sheath surrounding fascicles to maintain the blood-nerve barrier; and the endoneurium, which envelops individual nerve fibers and houses capillaries that nourish axons [11]. The endoneurium is the smallest unit visible on diagnostic imaging [12]. Functionally, these nerves are classified into motor nerves, which control muscle movement; sensory nerves, which relay tactile, pain, and temperature sensations; and autonomic nerves [13].

Nerve imaging biomarkers are classified into two main categories: anatomical and functional. Anatomical biomarkers, commonly assessed via ultrasound and MRI, evaluate nerve structure, with neuropathy diagnosis primarily relying on qualitative analysis. Functional biomarkers assess the physiological properties of nerves and muscles, providing insights into neuromuscular function and pathology, thereby enhancing sensitivity to early neuropathic changes [14].

The choice of imaging modality for PNP evaluation depends on the clinical context. Selection is tailored to the patient's medical history, laboratory results, and prior functional tests, ensuring a targeted and optimized diagnostic approach.

3. Imaging modalities in peripheral neuropathy

This subchapter begins with conventional imaging techniques and gradually explores advanced modalities, highlighting their advantages, limitations, and clinical diagnostic value.

3.1 Conventional radiography

Radiographs play a limited but valuable role in diagnosing potential nerve entrapment in compressive or post-traumatic peripheral neuropathy. While X-rays do not directly visualize nerves, they can reveal structural factors such as bone spurs, fractures, dislocation, callus, joint deformities, degenerative changes, foreign body, or soft tissue enlargement that may impinge on nerve pathways [15]. For example, a closed mid-shaft humeral fracture is associated with primary radial nerve neuropathy in approximately 10% of cases [16]. Bony abnormalities, such as exostoses, may impinge on adjacent nerves [17].

The X-ray evaluation of chronic peripheral neuropathy complications, particularly in diabetic foot disorders, aids in the detection of osteomyelitis, fractures, and structural deformities. In early stages, radiographs may reveal soft tissue swelling and subtle changes in adjacent fat, while advanced cases can show bone destruction, periosteal reactions, and sequestra formation indicative of chronic infection [18].

X-rays remain the primary imaging modality for the initial assessment of peripheral neuropathy. However, because soft tissues, including nerves and surrounding connective structures, are not well visualized, more advanced imaging techniques are often necessary for a definitive diagnosis of peripheral neuropathy.

3.2 Tomodensitometry

CT imaging usually serves as a complementary 3D modality to X-rays, providing enhanced visualization of bony abnormalities that may contribute to nerve injury and aiding in treatment planning [19]. It may serve as a valuable adjunct, particularly when combined with modalities like MRI and ultrasound. Angio-CT plays a role in detecting vascular anomalies, such as aneurysms that may compress the peripheral nerves [20]. The decision to utilize CT should be tailored to the patient's diagnostic hypothesis and/or clinician's specific needs ensuring a case-by-case approach for optimal diagnostic accuracy.

3.3 Ultrasound

The use of ultrasonography for assessing peripheral nerve lesions was first introduced in 1985 as a non-invasive imaging modality to evaluate nerve anatomy and pathology [21].

3.3.1 Morphological ultrasound

Ultrasound imaging is a safe, non-ionizing, cost-effective, and portable modality that enables real-time dynamic assessment of peripheral nerves. However, its diagnostic accuracy is operator-dependent, requiring advanced sonographic knowledge in anatomy. Optimizing peripheral nerve scanning requires selecting a high-frequency linear probe and adjusting the frequency, depth, and focus based on the nerve's anatomical location [22].

In regions accessible to sonography, targeted exam is the preferred imaging modality making it particularly valuable for assessing focal nerve injuries [23]. Advanced Doppler imaging further enhances the detection of tiny vascular structures and inflammation [24, 25]. Compared to clinical MRI, ultrasound provides superior spatial resolution, particularly due to the typically superficial location of peripheral nerves [26]. US demonstrates comparable specificity to MRI but offers higher sensitivity (93% vs. 67%) in detecting peripheral neuropathies [27].

Ultrasound protocols for peripheral nerve evaluation typically focus on assessing nerve morphology and continuity, measuring cross-sectional area and evaluating the surrounding soft tissue environment (**Table 1**). It allows for direct bilateral assessment, facilitating the detection of subtle asymmetries. Nerves typically appear as fascicular structures in the longitudinal plane and as honeycomb-like hypoechoic fascicles surrounded by a hyperechoic epineurium in the transverse plane. Compared to the adjacent structures, nerves are more echogenic than muscles but lesser so than tendons (**Figure 1**). This distinctive appearance enables differentiation from adjacent tendons, muscles, and vessels [23].

The pathologic presentation of nerve abnormalities evolves over time. In the acute phase, nerve injuries show accentuated fascicular pattern with swelling and hypoechogenicity and the interfascicular epineurium shows a thinned texture caused by fascicle swelling. Effacement of the normal structure as a diffusely hypoechoic nerve with inability to discern individual fascicles suggests neuropathy [12]. In the chronic phase, there is increased echogenicity and thickening of the epineurium and interfascicular soft tissue, accompanied by disruption of the fascicular architecture due to endoneurial fibrosis. Microcirculation is also affected, with low intra-fascicular vascularization in the acute phase due to capillary compression and increased extra-fascicular vascularization from epineurial vessel dilation. In the chronic phase, both intra- and extra-fascicular vascularization may increase due to endothelial hyperplasia and capillary ectasia [24, 28].

Feature	Key imaging questions	Considerations
Nerve Visibility and Swelling	Is the nerve visibly injured? Is it swollen(none/mild/moderate/severe)? What is the length of the affected segment?	Evaluate nerve morphology and signal changes.
Perineural Changes	Is there perineural fibrosis, hematoma, or inflammation? Is neural adhesion present? If fibrosis is present, what percentage of the neural circumference is affected?	Assess perineural tissue alterations and chronicity.
Neural Transection	Is there neural transection? If so, is it complete or incomplete?	Identify structural disruption and integrity.
Incomplete Transection	What percentage of the nerve is transected? What is the length of the gap (mm) between retracted fibers? Is fibrosis or neuroma-in-continuity (NIC) present? If so, what is its size?	Characterize residual neural continuity and reparative changes.
Complete Transection	What is the length of the gap (mm) between retracted nerve endings? Is there fibrosis or an end neuroma at the cut ends? If present, what is the neuroma size? What is the distance between the visibly normal nerve sections at either end of the transection?	Determine the severity of nerve discontinuity and potential for regeneration or surgical repair.

Table 1.
Systematic analysis of nerve injury characteristics in radiological evaluations.

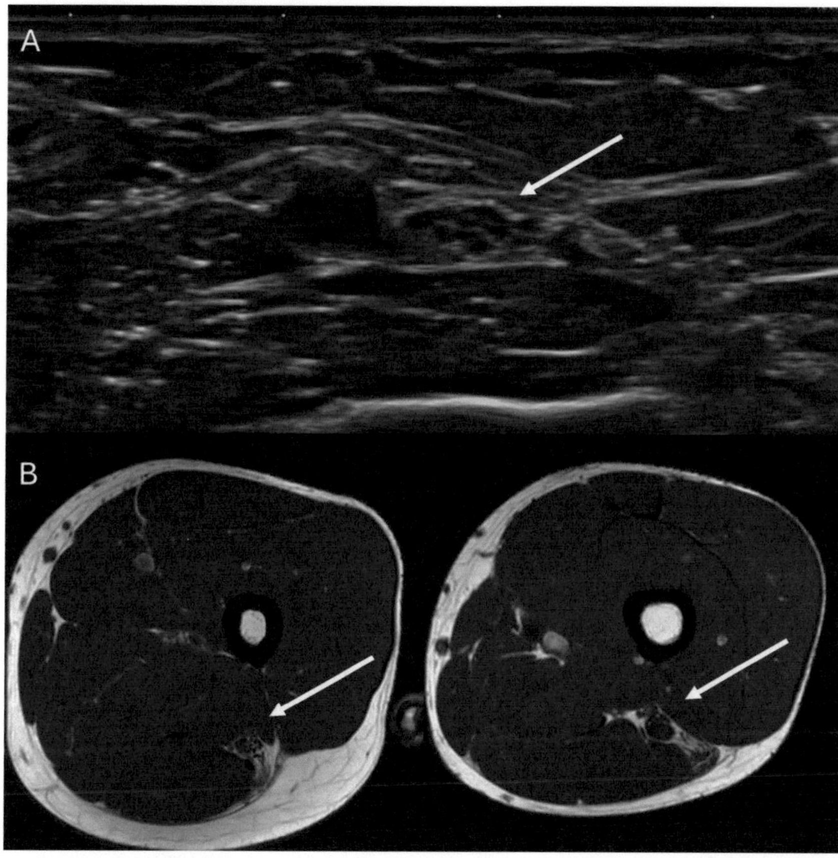

Figure 1.
(A) Illustrates the typical ultrasonographic appearance of median nerves in the transverse plane, they exhibit a honeycomb-like appearance, characterized by multiple hypoechoic fascicles embedded within a hyperechoic epineurium. This distinct echotexture aids in differentiating nerves from surrounding tissues in diagnostic imaging. (B) Illustrates the sciatic nerve in both normal and abnormal conditions on T1W sequence. On the left, the normal sciatic nerve exhibits a fascicular appearance with interfascicular fat visible between the fascicles. On the right, the abnormal sciatic nerve shows posterior fascicular thickening and loss of interfascicular fat, indicative of pathological changes.

3.3.2 Nerve elastography

Ultrasound elastography has emerged as a promising tool for assessing peripheral nerve pathology by providing quantitative data on nerve stiffness, which correlates with pathological changes in nerve composition. The technique, which includes strain elastography and shear wave elastography (SWE), has been extensively studied in conditions such as carpal tunnel syndrome, ulnar neuropathy, and diabetic peripheral neuropathy. Studies indicate that nerve stiffness increases in neuropathic conditions due to the replacement of compliant myelin with connective tissue. Despite its advantages, technical challenges such as standardization across ultrasound machines, limb positioning, and transducer orientation need to be addressed before it becomes a routine clinical tool [29].

3.3.3 Nerve quantitative ultrasound

More advanced quantitative ultrasound such as Backscattered radiofrequency (RF) signal characterization offers a method for assessing acoustic tissue properties, providing quantitative insights into tissue composition and microstructure. Parameters such as the backscatter coefficient and attenuation coefficient reflect tissue echogenicity and energy loss during wave propagation, correlating with histological features like collagen and myelin content. These techniques have been applied in evaluating nerves, with studies demonstrating significant correlations between RF-derived metrics and nerve pathology. However, limitations include artifacts, system-dependent variations, and depth-related signal degradation, particularly in vivo settings. Additionally, RF signal analysis often requires calibration with tissue-mimicking phantoms, increasing resource demands. While emerging methods seek to overcome these challenges through standardized calibration storage and advanced modeling, further refinement is needed to enhance its clinical applicability for peripheral nerve assessment [30].

3.3.4 Ultrasound limitation

A key limitation is the limited depth penetration and the complex anatomical course of peripheral nerves, which traverse multiple tissue planes. This complexity makes consistent evaluation challenging across different anatomical regions and patient morphotypes.

3.4 Magnetic resonance imaging

In the early 1990s, Filler and Howe's research group developed sequences with higher structural resolution and improved nerve lesion contrast, coining the term "Magnetic Resonance Neurography" (MRN) for this advanced imaging technique [31].

3.4.1 Morphological basic sequences

Imaging, particularly MRN, is usually reserved for atypical cases, including plexopathies, suspected malignancy, or unexplained neuropathic symptoms. MRN is a specialized MRI technique proven effective in evaluating and characterizing lesions affecting nerve roots, plexuses, and peripheral nerves.

High-field MRI (3 T) with thin slices and dedicated coils enables high-resolution, high-contrast 3D MRN, providing detailed visualization of the entire peripheral nerve along its axis while suppressing vascular signals, enhancing fascicular contrast, and characterizing perineural structures [32]. It can precisely identify the location and extent of nerve damage. Compared to ultrasound, MRI provides a more detailed visualization of nerve lesions in anatomically challenging regions. Additionally, its large field of view with superior contrast makes it more effective for assessing pathologies affecting multiple nerves and detecting muscle denervation [33, 34].

Like ultrasound, peripheral nerves are identified in transverse sections by their characteristic fascicular architecture. Pathological changes are detected through alterations in nerve morphology, including variations in shape, size, and contour, as well as changes in signal intensity [35].

High-resolution heavily T2-weighted (T2W 3D sequences with fat saturation) are essential. Normal nerve tissue appears isointense to surrounding muscle, but axonal injury leads to an increased intraneural T2 signal, detectable within 24–48 hours post-injury. This signal increase is observed not only at the lesion site but also along the distal nerve, reflecting Wallerian degeneration secondary to axonal damage [36]. An increase in T2W signal in nerves is a sensitive, though nonspecific, indicator of nerve injury. Further experiments revealed that trauma-induced T2W signal increases follow a proximal-to-distal gradient. Gradual normalization of the T2W signal, indicating nerve regeneration and motor recovery, also begins proximally at the lesion site and progresses distally. This breakthrough enabled the in vivo observation of nerve degeneration and regeneration [37].

T1-weighted (T1W) sequences are valuable for anatomical and morphological analysis, with high nerve-fat contrast, aiding in the identification of nerve abnormalities such as discontinuity, swelling, fat content, or compression-induced flattening (**Figure 1**).

Finally, normal muscle tissue shows an intermediate signal on T2W sequences, whereas an increased T2W signal may indicate muscle denervation, which can appear as early as five days after nerve injury [38]. T1W sequence can evaluate muscle fat involution, indicating chronic denervation [39].

3.4.2 Advanced sequences

Diffusion tensor imaging (DTI) and tractography are advanced MR imaging techniques that assess nerve structural connectivity and function [34]. DTI exploits the anisotropic nature of peripheral nerves, where water preferentially diffuses along the nerve axis, enabling the calculation of fractional anisotropy (FA) and apparent diffusion coefficient (ADC). FA reduction is associated with nerve injury, demyelination, and degeneration, while increased ADC suggests axonal damage. Tractography, a 3D reconstruction technique derived from DTI, visualizes nerve fiber pathways, aiding in nerve injury localization and surgical planning (**Figure 2**) [12].

The apparent T2 relaxation time (T2app) and proton spin density (ρ) are techniques used to quantify the T2W signal. T2app indicates endoneurial edema, while ρ reflects extracellular matrix changes, such as plasma protein leakage and inflammation. Applied successfully in hereditary transthyretin amyloidosis, T2app and ρ are promising biomarkers for peripheral nerve imaging [40].

Magnetization transfer contrast (MTC) imaging leverages the interaction between bound protons and free water molecules by using two nearly identical sequences: one with and one without an off-resonance saturation pulse. This allows for the calculation of the magnetization transfer ratio (MTR), which reflects the concentration of bound protons and their interaction with free water molecules. A change in the MTR reflects alterations in the concentration of macromolecules, particularly tissue proteins, providing indirect insights into the macromolecular composition and content of the tissue [41]. In chronic inflammatory demyelinating polyneuropathy (CIDP), magnetization transfer imaging (MTI) has shown a significantly reduced magnetization transfer ratio (MTR) ($p < 0.01$), indicating changes in macromolecular tissue composition. This reduction correlates significantly with electrophysiological markers of demyelination ($p < 0.05$) [42].

Healthy nerve tissue does not enhance with gadolinium-based contrast agents due to the intact blood-nerve barrier formed by the perineurium. Contrast-enhanced T1W sequences with fat saturation or subtraction techniques are useful for assessing inflammatory or infectious diseases, neoplasms, and excessive scar tissue formation in persistent or recurrent neuropathic symptoms post-decompression surgery [38].

Dynamic Contrast-Enhanced (DCE) MRI, capturing time-resolved images after the injection of a contrast agent, quantifies blood volume, vascular permeability, and

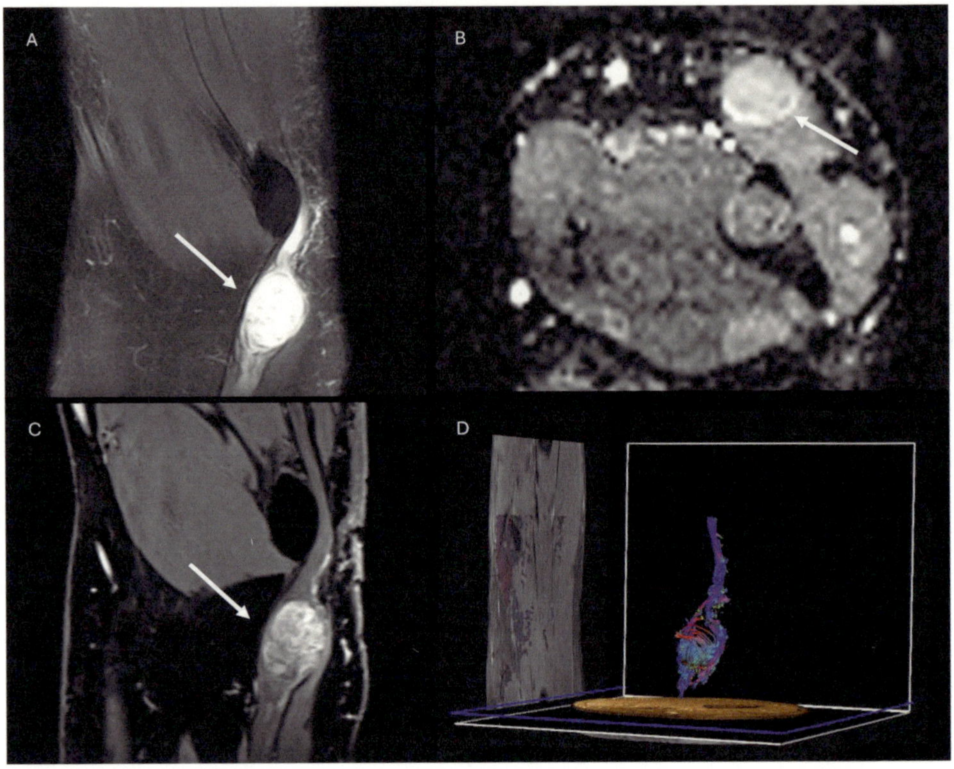

Figure 2.
53-year-old patient with an ulnar nerve schwannoma. (A) Sagittal T2-weighted fat-saturated MRI demonstrates a well-defined schwannoma along the ulnar nerve. (B) Axial ADC map imaging highlights no significative restriction. (C) Coronal 3D post-contrast T1 VIBE sequence illustrates the tumor's close relationship with the nerve along its trajectory. (D) Diffusion Tensor Imaging (DTI) tractography reveals nerve fiber displacement, demonstrating the schwannoma's mass effect on the ulnar nerve.

microcirculation [43]. Altered perfusion parameters correlate with nerve conduction abnormalities, particularly in diabetic neuropathy, where increased microvascular permeability is linked to nerve ischemia and disease progression [44]. Additionally, MR perfusion helps distinguish benign from malignant nerve tumors based on vascular patterns.

3.4.3 MRI limitations and pitfalls

MRI nerve imaging faces several practical challenges that impact diagnostic accuracy and feasibility. High costs, limited availability, and patient-related factors such as the need for prolonged stillness to minimize motion artifacts and claustrophobia can hinder its use. In extremities and small nerves, even slight movements degrade image quality, requiring patient compliance and longer acquisition times.

Technical constraints also affect diagnostic precision. While 3 T MRI improves resolution, it increases susceptibility artifacts, especially near air-bone interfaces, complicating nerve visualization. Fat suppression variability and the lack of standardized MR neurography (MRN) protocols further limit reproducibility and diagnostic consistency across institutions.

Interpretation remains challenging, as T2-weighted hyperintensities at physiological nerve constriction sites can mimic pathology [45]. The magic angle effect may falsely enhance nerve signal at specific limb positions [35], though its impact is reduced at 3 T [46]. In DTI analysis, age-related myelin loss lowers FA values, potentially mimicking neuropathy [47].

Despite advances in software and hardware, distinguishing true pathology from normal variations requires specialized radiology expertise, which is not widely available. Addressing these challenges calls for further protocol standardization, optimization of acquisition techniques, and increased subspecialized training to improve the clinical utility of MRI in peripheral nerve imaging [8].

3.5 Neuropathy score reporting and data system (NS-RADS)

The Neuropathy Score Reporting and Data System (NS-RADS) is an expert-validated standardized MRI reporting framework designed to improve the diagnosis, classification, and management of peripheral neuropathies such as BI-RADS in breast imaging.

It categorizes neuropathies based on cause, severity, and imaging characteristics, covering conditions such as nerve injury, entrapment, neoplasms, diffuse neuropathies, and post-intervention states. By integrating anatomical and functional imaging biomarkers, NS-RADS ensures a systematic and objective assessment of nerve abnormalities. Its reliability across different levels of radiology expertise makes it a valuable tool for clinical practice. This standardized approach facilitates multidisciplinary collaboration [48].

4. Clinical applications

The primary peripheral nerve pathologies prompting imaging referrals, ranked by frequency, include nerve entrapment syndromes, neoplastic lesions, traumatic nerve injuries, perineural fibrosis, neuralgic amyotrophy, and inflammatory neuropathies. These conditions are best assessed using high-resolution US or magnetic MRN, depending on the clinical context. Both modalities offer a complimentary detailed anatomical and pathological evaluation, aiding in accurate diagnosis [28]. This subchapter explores the key principles of PNP, where radiology plays a crucial role in patient management.

4.1 Traumatic peripheral nerve injuries

Traumatic peripheral nerve injuries occur due to penetrating wounds, crush injuries, or stretch injuries and are classified based on severity. Sunderland's classification expands on Seddon's system, categorizing nerve injuries from mild (neuropraxia) to severe (neurotmesis) (**Table 2**) [49]. MRN effectively detects nerve discontinuity, structural damage, neuromas, and denervation changes in muscles. Ultrasound is useful for real-time dynamic assessment and guiding interventions. Treatment varies based on the injury's type and severity. Complete nerve separation (neurotmesis) necessitates surgical intervention (nerve repair or grafting), and partial or incomplete nerve discontinuities (neuropraxia or axonotmesis) may recover spontaneously [50].

4.2 Compressive neuropathy

Nerves can be compressed as they pass through anatomical constraints such as myofascial planes or confined spaces like fibro-osseous or fibromuscular tunnels

Grade	Injured structures	US findings	MRI findings
1	Myelin	Normal or mildly hypoechoic nerve fascicles	Normal or T2 hyperintense nerve with or without muscle denervation
2	Myelin, axons	Enlarged, hypoechoic nerve fascicles	T2 hyperintense with or without mildly enlarged nerve plus muscle denervation
3	Myelin, axons, endoneurium	Enlarged, hypoechoic nerve	T2 hyperintense and enlarged nerve plus muscle denervation
4	Myelin, axons, endoneurium, perineurium	Enlarged, hypoechoic Nerve with intraneural scarring and potential focal enlargement (neuroma-in continuity)	Heterogeneous signal and enlarged nerve with disorganized/scarred fascicles, and potential focal enlargement (neuroma-in-continuity)
5	Myelin, axons, endoneurium, perineurium epineurium	Transection	Transection

Table 2.
Sunderland classification and US/MR corresponding semiology.

near joints. Enlargement of these tunnels' contents due to tumors, injuries, edema, hematomas, or repetitive muscle contractions can exacerbate nerve compression and compromise surrounding structures [47].

US and MRN have proven to be reliable imaging modalities for detecting pathologic alterations in chronic nerve entrapment syndromes or mass effect. Characteristic imaging findings include proximal and, occasionally, distal nerve swelling, with an abrupt caliber reduction and flattening at the compression site, known as the "notch" sign. Ultrasound reveals hypoechoic disruption of the normal fascicular "honeycomb" pattern, indicating structural disorganization [26]. On MRN, affected nerves exhibit conspicuous T2W hyperintensity adjacent to the compressive lesion, proximal fascicular enlargement, and, in severe cases, hyperintensity along the distal nerve course, reflecting Wallerian degeneration and denervated muscle changes [51]. Additionally, extrinsic compressive structures contributing to nerve entrapment are readily visualized on both imaging techniques (**Figure 3**).

US is highly effective for evaluating carpal tunnel and cubital tunnel syndromes due to its clear nerve visualization. It allows for precise cross-sectional measurements of the median nerve, helping assess nerve enlargement as it passes under the flexor retinaculum. A normal cross-sectional area (CSA) ranges between 9 and 11 mm^2, though the exact pathological threshold remains debated. One study found that a 2 mm^2 difference in CSA between the pronator quadratus level in the forearm and the carpal tunnel is highly sensitive and specific for carpal tunnel syndrome. Additional qualitative indicators include palmar bowing of the flexor retinaculum, nerve flattening, and a $\geq$ 30% enlargement of the nerve proximal to the retinaculum [52].

For cubital tunnel syndrome, the ulnar nerve is considered pathologically enlarged when its CSA exceeds 9 mm^2. A CSA ratio of $\geq$1,5:1 between the cubital tunnel and the proximal segment also suggests nerve enlargement. Dynamic US imaging can evaluate nerve subluxation, where the ulnar nerve moves out of the cubital tunnel and over the medial humeral epicondyle, which may cause symptoms [53].

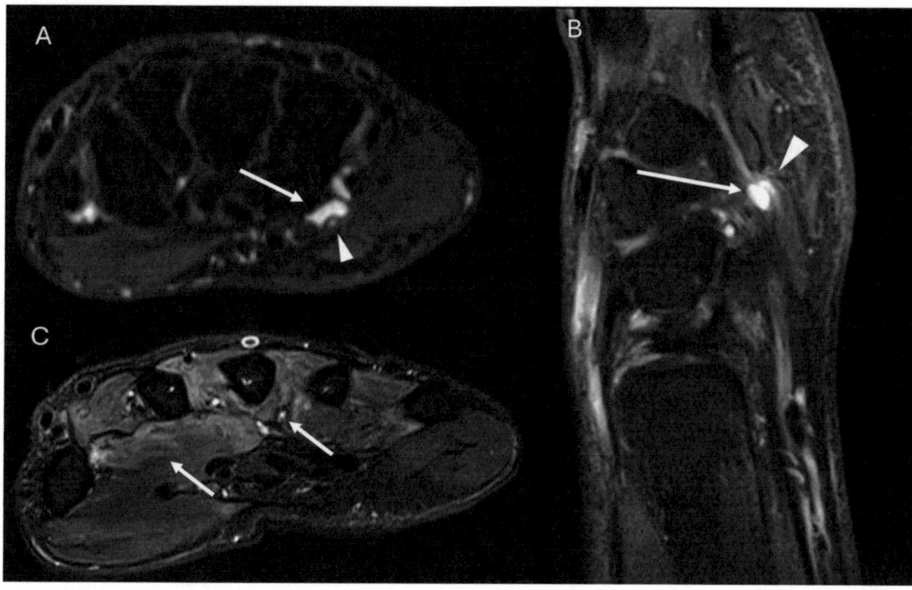

Figure 3.
Extrinsic compression of the motor branch of the ulnar nerve by a mucoid cyst. (A) Axial T2-weighted fat-saturated sequence demonstrates a mucoid cyst (arrow) in direct contact with the motor branch of the ulnar nerve (Arrowhead) at the level of the hamate bone. (B) Sagittal T2-weighted fat-saturated sequence confirms the cyst's mass effect and the ulnar nerve branch signal anomly (Arrowhead). (C) Axial DP fat-saturated sequence reveals denervation edema affecting the interosseous muscles and the adductor pollicis muscle, indicative of nerve compression-related muscle involvement.

4.3 Diabetes

The three most common etiologies of distal symmetric polyneuropathy are diabetes mellitus or impaired glucose tolerance, chronic alcohol consumption, and idiopathic causes [54].

The exact pathogenesis of diabetic peripheral neuropathy (DPN) remains debated, with two primary theories: the dying-back hypothesis, which suggests distal axonal degeneration progressing proximally, and the proximal nerve injury hypothesis, which proposes early damage at proximal nerve levels, particularly within the sciatic nerve [40, 55]. Histologically, DPN involves mixed axonal loss affecting both small and large fibers, leading to sensory deficits, pain, and motor dysfunction. MRN studies support the proximal nerve injury hypothesis, showing a proximal-to-distal lesion gradient in the sciatic nerve with clustered, multifocal lesions [56]. These findings align with prior histopathologic studies indicating ischemia-induced focal fiber loss [57].

Quantitative MRN markers further differentiate DPN from other neuropathies. An increase in proton spin density (ρ) suggests extracellular matrix alterations, while changes in T2 relaxation times reflect edema and structural nerve damage. Additionally, DPN pathology varies by diabetes type: Type 1 diabetes (T1D) is associated with T2 hyperintense lesions (indicating demyelination), whereas Type 2 diabetes (T2D) often shows T2 hypointense lesions, likely due to lipid accumulation [44]. Emerging evidence also highlights the role of dorsal root ganglia (DRG) degeneration in DPN progression, with decreased DRG volume correlating with symptom severity [58]. DTI studies further support FA reductions as an early marker of nerve damage [47, 59].

4.4 Hereditary transthyretin amyloidosis

Peripheral neuropathy in amyloidosis arises from amyloid fibril deposits impairing nerve function, particularly in hereditary transthyretin amyloidosis and systemic light chain amyloidosis. AL amyloidosis is caused by misfolded immunoglobulin light chains from plasma cell disorders and Hereditary Transthyretin Amyloidosis (ATTR) results from misfolded transthyretin (TTR) protein, either due to genetic mutations or age-related instability. This results in a progressive, length-dependent sensory-motor polyneuropathy, initially affecting small fibers and causing pain and numbness in the feet before spreading to larger myelinated fibers [60].

MRN studies identify diffuse, proximally dominant nerve lesions, distinguishing amyloidosis from the multifocal pattern seen in diabetic neuropathy. Early nerve damage is marked by increased proton spin density (ρ), indicating amyloid-related extracellular matrix alterations, while elevated T2 relaxation time (T2app) in later stages suggests endoneurial edema and nerve degeneration [40].

The sciatic nerve magnetization transfer ratio (MTR) correlates with disease severity, reflecting progressive axonal damage. Importantly, MRN can detect nerve abnormalities before symptoms appear, facilitating early diagnosis, especially in asymptomatic variant ATTR carriers. Additionally, while both ATTR and Light chain amyloidosis exhibit proximal lesion predominance, ATTR presents earlier and more diffusely [61]. MRN is a valuable non-invasive biomarker for early detection and disease monitoring, particularly with emerging treatments like TTR stabilizers and RNA-based therapies [62, 63].

4.5 Inflammatory/immune peripheral neuropathy

Guillain–Barré Syndrome (GBS) and Acute-Onset Chronic Inflammatory Demyelinating Polyradiculoneuritis (CIDP) are both immune-mediated peripheral neuropathies that primarily affect the myelin sheath and nerve roots, leading to progressive motor and sensory deficits. GBS is an acute, rapidly progressive disorder that often follows a viral or bacterial infection, triggering an autoimmune attack on peripheral nerves. It typically presents with ascending weakness, areflexia, sensory disturbances, and autonomic dysfunction. GBS is usually monophasic and self-limiting, with many patients recovering with intravenous immunoglobulin or plasma exchange [64]. CIDP, on the other hand, is a chronic and relapsing neuropathy with a more prolonged course. While some CIDP cases may present acutely, the disease progresses beyond eight weeks, often requiring long-term immunotherapy such as IVIG, corticosteroids, or plasma exchange. CIDP leads to progressive demyelination and axonal damage, resulting in persistent motor weakness, sensory loss, and functional disability [65].

Imaging plays a role in differentiating GBS and acute-onset CIDP, two immune-mediated neuropathies with overlapping early clinical presentations but distinct treatment courses. In GBS, characteristic findings include nerve root and vagus nerve enlargement, while sensory nerves remain unaffected. In contrast, CIDP exhibits multifocal nerve enlargement, particularly involving both sensory and sensorimotor nerves, often persisting beyond six months with signs of fibrosis.

Longitudinal imaging follow-up further aids in monitoring disease evolution. In GBS, nerve enlargement typically resolves within six months, supporting its self-limiting course, while in CIDP, persistent nerve hypertrophy and increased echointensity indicate ongoing chronic nerve damage. This distinction is vital, as GBS usually requires a single round of intravenous immunoglobulin or plasma exchange, whereas CIDP often necessitates prolonged immunotherapy. By combining with electrodiagnostic data, imaging enhances early diagnosis and prognosis estimation [65].

4.6 Peripheral nerve sheath tumors

Peripheral nerve sheath tumors (PNSTs) include benign variants, such as schwannomas and neurofibromas, and malignant peripheral nerve sheath tumors (MPNSTs), which require early detection. Schwannomas are well-defined, encapsulated tumors that displace nerve fascicles, appearing T2W hyperintense on MRN with gadolinium enhancement, while ultrasound shows a hypoechoic, well-circumscribed mass. Neurofibromas, often associated with NF1, infiltrate the nerve and may exhibit a T2W "target sign" on MRN due to central fibrosis, whereas ultrasound shows diffuse nerve enlargement with fascicular disruption. MPNSTs, aggressive malignant tumors, are characterized by large size (>5 cm), ill-defined margins, heterogeneous enhancement, and perilesional edema [66].

MRN plays a crucial role in diagnosing and characterizing peripheral nerve tumors by utilizing DWI and DTI. DWI, through ADC mapping, helps distinguish benign from malignant tumors, with benign tumors showing higher ADC values, whereas malignant peripheral nerve sheath tumors typically exhibit lower ADC due to high cellularity and restricted diffusion. Whole-body DWI is a highly effective screening tool for systemic disorders like NF1 and Li-Fraumeni syndrome, enabling the detection of potentially malignant lesions characterized by diffusion restriction [67].

DTI, which measures both the magnitude and direction of water diffusion, provides additional insights into nerve integrity through FA and tractography, which assess fiber continuity and nerve displacement (**Figure 2**). These techniques are particularly useful for evaluating tumor-induced nerve compression, degeneration, or infiltration which can aid in surgical planning by identifying nerve fibers within or adjacent to tumors, helping to preserve nerve function during resection. Ultrasound aids in real-time evaluation and biopsy guidance. Finally, perfusion imaging further assists in monitoring tumor progression and distinguishing recurrent tumors from post-treatment fibrosis [8].

4.7 Nerve tumor infiltration

Peripheral nerves can be infiltrated by various malignant tumors, either through direct invasion, perineural spread, or metastatic involvement. Among the most common malignancies that affect peripheral nerves are lymphomas, breast cancer, lung cancer, prostate cancer, colorectal cancer, and head and neck tumors.

MRI with gadolinium contrast is the first-line modality for detecting structural nerve abnormalities, but it can be challenging to interpret in post-surgical or post-radiation settings. FDG-PET/CT complements MRI by differentiating benign post-treatment changes from active malignancy, guiding biopsy site selection, and assessing tumor metabolism and treatment response [68].

Neurolymphomatosis, the infiltration of nerves by lymphoma cells, typically presents as fusiform nerve enlargement, increased T2W signal intensity, and diffuse contrast enhancement. Perineural spread, commonly seen in head and neck cancers, as well as prostate and breast cancer, manifests as nodular nerve thickening with abnormal enhancement. Radiation-induced plexopathy, often occurring after treatment, must be distinguished from tumor recurrence, as it presents with nerve thickening and mild enhancement but minimal FDG uptake at TEP scan compared to malignant lesions. Imaging plays a critical role in the diagnosis, treatment planning, and follow-up of nerve infiltrating tumors. The combination of anatomical and functional imaging improves diagnostic accuracy [69].

4.8 Leprosy

Leprosy is a chronic infectious neuropathy caused by *Mycobacterium leprae*, primarily affecting the skin and peripheral nerve due to the unique affinity for Schwann cells. The disease leads to progressive sensory loss, increasing the risk of trauma, infections, and ultimately nerve damage and deformities. Clinically, leprosy presents in a spectrum ranging from tuberculoid to lepromatous forms, with borderline subtypes exhibiting intermediate features. Nerve involvement is common and may lead to enlargement, fibrosis, and functional impairment, particularly in the ulnar, median, and posterior tibial nerves. US and MRI are valuable tools in evaluating leprosy neuropathy. Affected nerves often appear enlarged, with abnormal fascicular patterns. US reveals fusiform nerve swelling, loss of fascicular architecture, and hypoechoic changes, while Doppler US may detect increased endoneurial blood

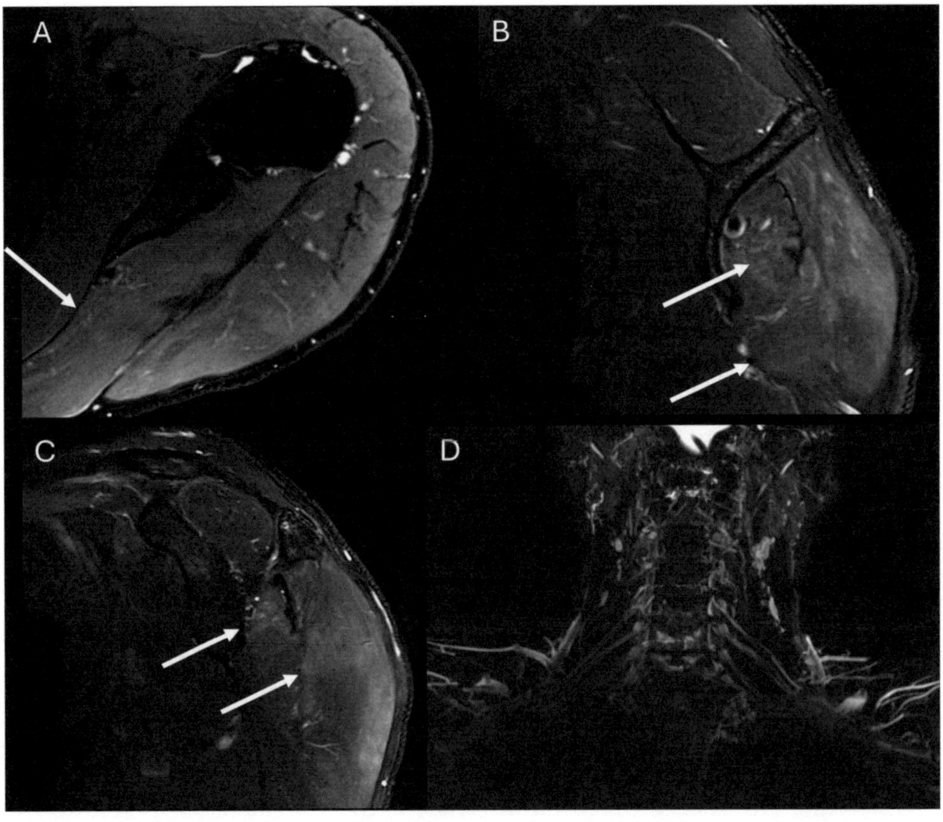

Figure 4.
A 32-year-old patient with post-viral Parsonage-Turner syndrome. (A) Axial T2-weighted fat-saturated MRI demonstrates a heterogeneous intermediate signal alteration in the posterior deltoid and infraspinatus muscles. (B, C) Coronal T2-weighted fat-saturated MRI further reveals a heterogeneous intermediate signal abnormality involving the infraspinatus, teres minor, and posterior deltoid muscles. (D) MRI of the brachial plexus shows no signal abnormality.

flow, indicating active neuritis. MRI findings include T2W hyperintensity, gadolinium enhancement, and nerve thickening, especially during reversal reactions and erythema nodosum leprosum episodes [70].

4.9 Parsonage turner

Parsonage turner (PTS), also known as acute idiopathic brachial plexus neuritis, is a rare inflammatory neuropathy affecting the brachial plexus, leading to severe shoulder pain followed by muscle weakness and atrophy. It is often preceded by infections, vaccinations, or surgery and primarily affects the C5 and upper trunk of the brachial plexus. MRN is the preferred imaging modality for evaluating PTS, allowing direct visualization of nerve abnormalities and muscle denervation. MRN findings typically show T2 hyperintensity and mild thickening in the affected nerves, predominantly involving the roots, trunks, and cords. In the acute phase, MRN reveals muscle edema, while the chronic phase is characterized by fatty infiltration and atrophy, particularly in the supraspinatus and infraspinatus muscles. MRN aids in ruling out alternative causes (e.g., cervical radiculopathy, rotator cuff pathology) and in confirming the diagnosis (**Figure 4**) [71].

5. Imaging-guided interventional applications

5.1 Peripheral nerve blocks and infiltration

Studies indicate that ultrasound-guided peripheral nerve blocks (PNBs), either independently or in conjunction with peripheral nerve stimulation, demonstrate superior efficacy in achieving enhanced sensory and motor blockade, minimizing the need for supplemental anesthesia, and reducing the incidence of minor procedural complications [9]. Perineural infiltration for pain management involves the targeted administration of local anesthetics, corticosteroids, adhesiolysis agents, and neuromuscular blockers to alleviate neuropathic pain and inflammation. Lidocaine and bupivacaine are commonly used for diagnostic and therapeutic nerve blocks. Dexamethasone is frequently added to enhance the anti-inflammatory effects and prolong nerve block duration without significant adverse effects. The procedure is generally safe, with complications being rare and transient. To minimize risks such as nerve injury, local anesthetic toxicity, allergic reactions, and infection, strict aseptic techniques, imaging guidance (CT or ultrasound), and careful needle placement are essential [72].

5.2 Radiofrequency

Radiofrequency ablation (RFA) is an effective, minimally invasive procedure used for chronic peripheral nerve pain when conservative treatments fail. It works by using thermal energy or pulsed electromagnetic fields to create a controlled lesion on sensory nerves, disrupting pain signals while preserving motor function. RFA is widely applied to major joint-related pain syndromes such as knee (genicular nerve ablation) offering sustained relief in osteoarthritis and degenerative conditions. It is also effective in treating neuropathies, including trigeminal neuralgia; ilioinguinal, iliohypogastric, and genitofemoral neuralgia; meralgia paresthetica; and pudendal neuralgia, providing long-term pain reduction. The procedure is safe and well-tolerated, with minor complications like transient discomfort and a low risk of nerve damage. Emerging advanced techniques, such as cooled and pulsed RFA, enhance precision and safety, making RFA a viable alternative to long-term opioid use or surgical intervention for chronic pain syndromes [73].

5.3 Cryoablation

Cryoneurolysis is an interventional technique that applies extreme cold to sensory nerves, leading to prolonged analgesia by inducing Wallerian degeneration while preserving the myelin sheath and endoneurium. This method is performed under ultrasound or CT guidance forming an ice ball capable of disrupting nerve conduction. The procedure is optimized for chronic pain management, including peripheral neuropathies, post-surgical pain syndromes, phantom limb pain, low back pain, and metastatic bone pain. Its advantages include a lower risk of neuritis, neuroma formation, and motor impairment, making it a viable alternative for long-term pain relief (**Figure 5**) [74].

5.4 Biopsy

Ultrasound-guided core needle biopsy is a highly accurate and safe diagnostic tool for evaluating PNSTs. It offers a minimally invasive alternative to incisional biopsy, with a diagnostic accuracy of 99.3%, high sensitivity (90.9%), and specificity (100%), making it reliable for distinguishing benign from malignant PNSTs. Additionally, it has a low complication rate. The procedure is cost-effective, faster

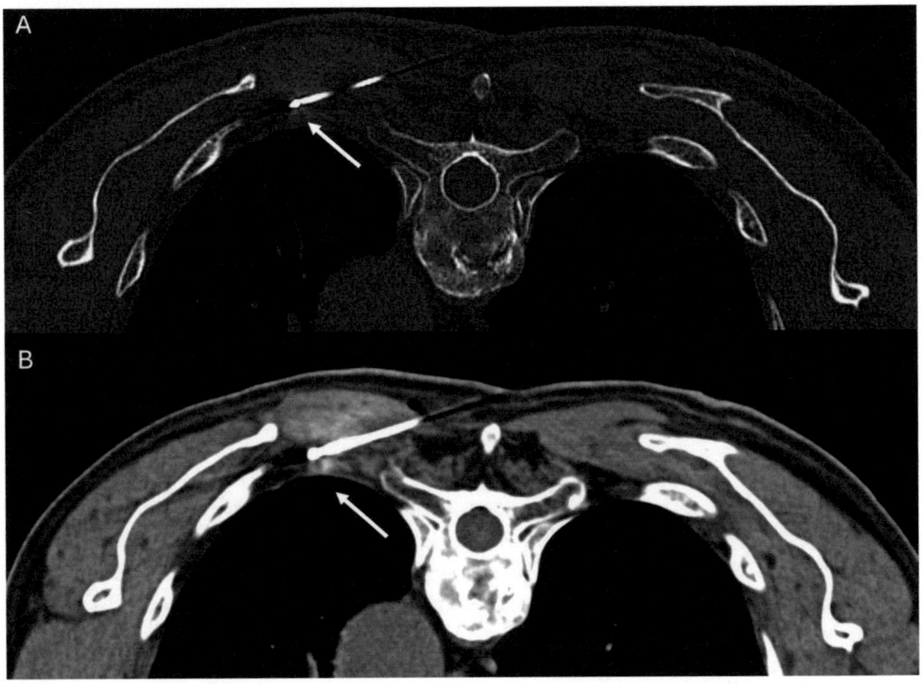

Figure 5.
CT-guided cryoablation of the left T5 intercostal nerve in a patient suffering from neuropathic pain following herpes zoster. (A): Bone window. (B): Soft tissue window.

than traditional surgical biopsies, and minimizes the risk of tumor cell contamination, making it a preferred method for diagnosing nerve tumors [10].

5.5 Carpal tunnel release

Ultrasound-guided percutaneous carpal tunnel release is a minimally invasive technique that uses real-time ultrasound to safely transect the transverse carpal ligament while avoiding nerve and vascular injury [75]. Studies report significant symptom relief as early as one week, with faster recovery (return to work in 4–5 days vs. 26 days for mini-open techniques). Ultrasound confirms median nerve decompression with rare complications. Based on very low level of evidence, this technique offers faster recovery, less pain, and fewer complications than traditional surgery, though further studies are needed for long-term validation [76].

5.6 Platelet-rich plasma injection

Platelet-Rich Plasma (PRP) has demonstrated promising regenerative effects in peripheral nerve injuries by enhancing axon regrowth, Schwann cell activation, and vascularization. PRP contains bioactive growth factors such as VEGF, PDGF, and IGF-1, which stimulate angiogenesis, neuroprotection, and anti-inflammatory responses [77]. Studies indicate that PRP reduces neuronal apoptosis, modulates the inflammatory microenvironment by promoting macrophage polarization, and facilitates Schwann cell migration and proliferation, which are crucial for nerve repair. In clinical applications, ultrasound-guided PRP injections have shown improved functional recovery in conditions like carpal tunnel syndrome and traumatic nerve injuries [78]. While results are promising, standardization of PRP preparation remains a challenge, and further clinical trials are needed to optimize protocols and confirm long-term safety and efficacy [79].

5.7 Stem cell therapy

The localized application of stem cell therapy represents a promising strategy for treating peripheral nerve injuries, leveraging its regenerative, neuroprotective, and anti-inflammatory effects. Mesenchymal stem cells derived from bone marrow, adipose tissue, dental pulp, umbilical cord, or amniotic fluid are particularly effective as they can differentiate into Schwann-like cells, secrete neurotrophic factors (e.g., NGF, BDNF, GDNF), and enhance axon regeneration. These cells promote myelination, reduce apoptosis, and modulate immune responses, thereby creating a favorable microenvironment for nerve repair. Stem cell secretome, which includes exosomes and growth factors, also plays a crucial role in nerve regeneration by stimulating axonal elongation and Schwann cell migration. Moreover, MSCs can be combined with biomaterial nerve conduits to improve scaffold-based nerve regeneration. While preclinical and clinical studies show promising results, challenges remain regarding optimal cell source, delivery methods, and long-term safety, necessitating further research to refine this approach for widespread clinical application [50].

6. Conclusion

Radiology has become a pivotal tool in the evaluation and management of peripheral neuropathy. Although imaging alone cannot establish the etiology of neuropathy, which remains dependent on the clinical context, it provides a more comprehensive and precise assessment by delineating anatomical abnormalities and identifying pathological changes. As technology advances, multimodal advanced imaging becomes indispensable for complex peripheral neuropathy, revolutionizing both diagnostic and treatment strategies.

Funding

This article review did not receive any specific grant from funding agencies in the public, commercial, or not-for-profit sectors.

Declaration competing interests

The authors declare that they have no competing interests.

Ethical approval

This article review does not contain any studies with human participants or animals performed by any of the authors.

Consent to participate

Not applicable. This study does not involve human participants requiring consent.

Consent to publish

Not applicable. The manuscript does not include any individual person's data in any form requiring consent.

Acronym

US	ultrasound
MRI	magnetic resonance imaging
MRN	magnetic resonance neurography
PNP	peripheral neuropathy
DWI	diffusion-weighted imaging
DTI	diffusion tensor imaging
ADC	apparent diffusion coefficient
FA	fractional anisotropy

Author details

Salim Zenkhri
Department of Radiology, University of Montreal Hospital Center (CHUM), Montreal, QC, Canada

*Address all correspondence to: salim.zenkhri@gmail.com

References

[1] Martyn CN, Hughes RA. Epidemiology of peripheral neuropathy. Journal of Neurology, Neurosurgery, and Psychiatry. 1997;**62**:310-318

[2] New horizons in diabetic neuropathy: Mechanisms, bioenergetics, and pain - PMC n.d. https://pmc.ncbi.nlm.nih.gov/articles/PMC5400015/ [Accessed: January 17, 2025]

[3] Hanewinckel R, Drenthen J, van Oijen M, Hofman A, van Doorn PA, Ikram MA. Prevalence of polyneuropathy in the general middle-aged and elderly population. Neurology. 2016;**87**:1892-1898. DOI: 10.1212/WNL.0000000000003293

[4] Hanewinckel R, van Oijen M, Ikram MA, van Doorn PA. The epidemiology and risk factors of chronic polyneuropathy. European Journal of Epidemiology. 2016;**31**:5-20. DOI: 10.1007/s10654-015-0094-6

[5] Castelli G, Desai KM, Cantone RE. Peripheral neuropathy: Evaluation and differential diagnosis. American Family Physician. 2020;**102**:732-739

[6] Dyck PJ, Oviatt KF, Lambert EH. Intensive evaluation of referred unclassified neuropathies yields improved diagnosis. Annals of Neurology. 1981;**10**:222-226. DOI: 10.1002/ana.410100304

[7] Stewart JD. Peripheral nerve fascicles: Anatomy and clinical relevance. Muscle & Nerve. 2003;**28**:525-541. DOI: 10.1002/mus.10454

[8] Eajazi A, Weinschenk C, Chhabra A. Imaging biomarkers of peripheral nerves: Focus on magnetic resonance neurography and ultrasonography. Seminars in Musculoskeletal Radiology. 2024;**28**:92-102. DOI: 10.1055/s-0043-1776427

[9] Lewis SR, Price A, Walker KJ, McGrattan K, Smith AF. Ultrasound guidance for upper and lower limb blocks. Cochrane Database of Systematic Reviews. 2015;**2015**:CD006459. DOI: 10.1002/14651858.CD006459.pub3

[10] Tøttrup M, Eriksen JD, Hellfritzsch MB, Sørensen FB, Baad-Hansen T. Diagnostic accuracy of ultrasound-guided core biopsy of peripheral nerve sheath tumors. Journal of Clinical Ultrasound. 2020;**48**:134-138. DOI: 10.1002/jcu.22769

[11] Menorca RMG, Fussell TS, Elfar JC. Nerve physiology: Mechanisms of injury and recovery. Hand Clinics. 2013;**29**:317-330. DOI: 10.1016/j.hcl.2013.04.002

[12] Holzgrefe RE, Wagner ER, Singer AD, Daly CA. Imaging of the peripheral nerve: Concepts and future direction of magnetic resonance neurography and ultrasound. Journal of Hand Surgery. 2019;**44**:1066-1079. DOI: 10.1016/j.jhsa.2019.06.021

[13] Lundborg G, Dahlin LB. Anatomy, function, and pathophysiology of peripheral nerves and nerve compression. Hand Clinics. 1996;**12**:185-193. DOI: 10.1016/S0749-0712(21)00303-6

[14] Chhabra A, Chalian M, Soldatos T, Andreisek G, Faridian-Aragh N, Williams E, et al. 3-T high-resolution MR neurography of sciatic neuropathy. AJR. American Journal of Roentgenology. 2012;**198**:W357-W364. DOI: 10.2214/AJR.11.6981

[15] Hochman MG, Zilberfarb JL. Nerves in a pinch: Imaging of nerve compression syndromes. Radiologia Clinica. 2004;**42**:221-245. DOI: 10.1016/S0033-8389(03)00162-3

[16] Hendrickx LAM, Hilgersom NFJ, Alkaduhimi H, Doornberg JN, van den Bekerom MPJ. Radial nerve palsy associated with closed humeral shaft fractures: A systematic review of 1758 patients. Archives of Orthopaedic and Trauma Surgery. 2021;**141**:561-568. DOI: 10.1007/s00402-020-03446-y

[17] Göçmen S, Topuz AK, Atabey C, Şimşek H, Keklikçi K, Rodop O. Peripheral nerve injuries due to osteochondromas: Analysis of 20 cases and review of the literature. Journal of Neurosurgery. 2014;**120**(5):1105-1112. DOI: 10.3171/2013.11.JNS13310

[18] Daneshvar K, Anwander H. Diagnostic imaging of diabetic foot disorders. Foot and Ankle Clinics. 2022;**27**:513-527. DOI: 10.1016/j.fcl.2022.01.002

[19] van den Hurk L, van den Besselaar M, Scheltinga M. Exercise induced neuropathic lower leg pain due to a tibial bone exostosis. The Physician and Sportsmedicine. 2021;**49**:363-366. DOI: 10.1080/00913847.2021.1910006

[20] Zied M, Farouk C, Mohsen C, Wajdi C, Ali H, Wael G. Guyon's canal syndrome resulting from an ulnar artery aneurysm: A case report. International Journal of Surgery Case Reports. 2024;**121**:109978. DOI: 10.1016/j.ijscr.2024.109978

[21] Solbiati L, De Pra L, Ierace T, Bellotti E, Derchi L. High-resolution sonography of the recurrent laryngeal nerve: Anatomic and pathologic considerations. American Journal of Roentgenology. 1985;**145**:989-993. DOI: 10.2214/ajr.145.5.989

[22] Ricci V, Abdulsalam AJ, Özçakar L. Ultrasound imaging for dummies: Getting oriented among the planes. Journal of Rehabilitation Medicine. 2019;**51**:624-625. DOI: 10.2340/16501977-2581

[23] Albano D, Aringhieri G, Messina C, De Flaviis L, Sconfienza LM. High-frequency and ultra-high frequency ultrasound: Musculoskeletal imaging up to 70 MHz. Seminars in Musculoskeletal Radiology. 2020;**24**:125-134. DOI: 10.1055/s-0039-3401042

[24] Ricci V, Ricci C, Cocco G, Gervasoni F, Donati D, Farì G, et al. Histopathology and high-resolution ultrasound imaging for peripheral nerve (injuries). Journal of Neurology. 2022;**269**:3663-3675. DOI: 10.1007/s00415-022-10988-1

[25] Dong Y, Alhaskawi A, Zhou H, Zou X, Liu Z, Ezzi SHA, et al. Imaging diagnosis in peripheral nerve injury. Frontiers in Neurology. 2023;**14**. DOI: 10.3389/fneur.2023.1250808

[26] Ali ZS, Pisapia JM, Ma TS, Zager EL, Heuer GG, Khoury V. Ultrasonographic evaluation of peripheral nerves. World Neurosurgery. 2016;**85**:333-339. DOI: 10.1016/j.wneu.2015.10.005

[27] Zaidman CM, Seelig MJ, Baker JC, Mackinnon SE, Pestronk A. Detection of peripheral nerve pathology: Comparison of ultrasound and MRI. Neurology. 2013;**80**:1634-1640. DOI: 10.1212/WNL.0b013e3182904f3f

[28] Griffith JF, Guggenberger R. Peripheral nerve imaging. In: Hodler J, Kubik-Huch RA, von Schulthess GK, editors. Musculoskelet. Dis. 2021-2024

Diagn. Imaging. Cham (CH): Springer; 2021

[29] Wee TC, Simon NG. Ultrasound elastography for the evaluation of peripheral nerves: A systematic review. Muscle & Nerve. 2019;**60**:501-512. DOI: 10.1002/mus.26624

[30] Jerban S, Barrère V, Andre M, Chang EY, Shah SB. Quantitative ultrasound techniques used for peripheral nerve assessment. Diagnostics. 2023;**13**:956. DOI: 10.3390/diagnostics13050956

[31] Filler AG, Howe FA, Hayes CE, Kliot M, Winn HR, Bell BA, et al. Magnetic resonance neurography. Lancet Lond Engl. 1993;**341**:659-661. DOI: 10.1016/0140-6736(93)90422-d

[32] Bischoff C, Kollmer J, Schulte-Mattler W. State-of-the-art diagnosis of peripheral nerve trauma: clinical examination, electrodiagnostic, and imaging. In: Mod. Concepts Peripher. Nerve Repair. 2017. pp. 11-25

[33] Aagaard BD, Maravilla KR, Kliot M. Magnetic resonance neurography: Magnetic resonance imaging of peripheral nerves. Neuroimaging Clinics of North America. 2001;**11**(viii):131-146

[34] Chen Y, Haacke EM, Li J. Peripheral nerve magnetic resonance imaging. F1000Research. 2019;**8**:F1000 Faculty Rev-1803. DOI: 10.12688/f1000research.19695.1

[35] Chappell KE, Robson MD, Stonebridge-Foster A, Glover A, Allsop JM, Williams AD, et al. Magic angle effects in MR neurography. American Journal of Neuroradiology. 2004;**25**:431-440

[36] Filler AG, Kliot M, Howe FA, Hayes CE, Saunders DE, Goodkin R, et al. Application of magnetic resonance neurography in the evaluation of patients with peripheral nerve pathology. Journal of Neurosurgery. 1996;**85**:299-309. DOI: 10.3171/jns.1996.85.2.0299

[37] Bendszus M, Wessig C, Solymosi L, Reiners K, Koltzenburg M. MRI of peripheral nerve degeneration and regeneration: Correlation with electrophysiology and histology. Experimental Neurology. 2004;**188**:171-177. DOI: 10.1016/j.expneurol.2004.03.025

[38] West GA, Haynor DR, Goodkin R, Tsuruda JS, Bronstein AD, Kraft G, et al. Magnetic resonance imaging signal changes in denervated muscles after peripheral nerve injury. Neurosurgery. 1994;**35**:1077-1085; discussion 1085-1086. DOI: 10.1227/00006123-199412000-00010

[39] Yang Y, Qiu L, Gu X, Chen J, Chen S, Hu D, et al. Monitoring rotator cuff muscle fatty infiltration progression by magnetic resonance imaging T1 mapping: Correlation with direct evaluation findings in rats. The American Journal of Sports Medicine. 2022;**50**:1078-1087. DOI: 10.1177/03635465211069976

[40] Kollmer J, Hund E, Hornung B, Hegenbart U, Schönland SO, Kimmich C, et al. In vivo detection of nerve injury in familial amyloid polyneuropathy by magnetic resonance neurography. Brain: A Journal of Neurology. 2015;**138**:549-562. DOI: 10.1093/brain/awu344

[41] Wolff SD, Balaban RS. Magnetization transfer contrast (MTC) and tissue water proton relaxation in vivo. Magnetic Resonance in Medicine. 1989;**10**:135-144. DOI: 10.1002/mrm.1910100113

[42] Preisner F, Pitarokoili K, Lueling B, Motte J, Fisse AL, Grüter T, et al. Quantitative magnetic resonance neurography in chronic inflammatory demyelinating polyradiculoneuropathy: A longitudinal study over 6 years. Annals of Clinical Translational Neurology. 2024;**11**:593-606. DOI: 10.1002/acn3.51978

[43] Bäumer P, Reimann M, Decker C, Radbruch A, Bendszus M, Heiland S, et al. Peripheral nerve perfusion by dynamic contrast-enhanced magnetic resonance imaging: Demonstration of feasibility. Investigative Radiology. 2014;**49**:518-523. DOI: 10.1097/RLI.0000000000000046

[44] Jende JME, Groener JB, Oikonomou D, Heiland S, Kopf S, Pham M, et al. Diabetic neuropathy differs between type 1 and type 2 diabetes: Insights from magnetic resonance neurography. Annals of Neurology. 2018;**83**:588-598. DOI: 10.1002/ana.25182

[45] Husarik DB, Saupe N, Pfirrmann CWA, Jost B, Hodler J, Zanetti M. Elbow nerves: MR findings in 60 asymptomatic subjects--Normal anatomy, variants, and pitfalls. Radiology. 2009;**252**:148-156. DOI: 10.1148/radiol.2521081614

[46] Kästel T, Heiland S, Bäumer P, Bartsch AJ, Bendszus M, Pham M. Magic angle effect: A relevant artifact in MR neurography at 3T? AJNR. American Journal of Neuroradiology. 2011;**32**:821-827. DOI: 10.3174/ajnr.A2402

[47] Kollmer J, Bendszus M. Magnetic resonance neurography: Improved diagnosis of peripheral neuropathies. Neurotherapeutics. 2021;**18**:2368-2383. DOI: 10.1007/s13311-021-01166-8

[48] Chhabra A, Deshmukh SD, Lutz AM, Fritz J, Sneag DB, Mogharrabi B, et al. Neuropathy score reporting and data system (NS-RADS): MRI reporting guideline of peripheral neuropathy explained and reviewed. Skeletal Radiology. 2022;**51**:1909-1922. DOI: 10.1007/s00256-022-04061-1

[49] Sunderland S. A classification of peripheral nerve injuries producing loss of function. Brain: A Journal of Neurology. 1951;**74**:491-516. DOI: 10.1093/brain/74.4.491

[50] Lopes B, Sousa P, Alvites R, Branquinho M, Sousa AC, Mendonça C, et al. Peripheral nerve injury treatments and advances: One health perspective. International Journal of Molecular Sciences. 2022;**23**:918. DOI: 10.3390/ijms23020918

[51] Chhabra A, Madhuranthakam AJ, Andreisek G. Magnetic resonance neurography: Current perspectives and literature review. European Radiology. 2018;**28**:698-707. DOI: 10.1007/s00330-017-4976-8

[52] Cartwright MS, Hobson-Webb LD, Boon AJ, Alter KE, Hunt CH, Flores VH, et al. Evidence-based guideline: Neuromuscular ultrasound for the diagnosis of carpal tunnel syndrome. Muscle & Nerve. 2012;**46**:287-293. DOI: 10.1002/mus.23389

[53] Chen I-J, Chang K-V, Wu W-T, Özçakar L. Ultrasound parameters other than the direct measurement of ulnar nerve size for diagnosing cubital tunnel syndrome: A systemic review and meta-analysis. Archives of Physical Medicine and Rehabilitation. 2019;**100**:1114-1130. DOI: 10.1016/j.apmr.2018.06.021

[54] Eleftheriadou A, Williams S, Nevitt S, Brown E, Roylance R, Wilding JPH, et al. The prevalence

of cardiac autonomic neuropathy in prediabetes: A systematic review. Diabetologia. 2021;**64**:288-303. DOI: 10.1007/s00125-020-05316-z

[55] Behse F, Buchthal F, Carlsen F. Nerve biopsy and conduction studies in diabetic neuropathy. Journal of Neurology, Neurosurgery, and Psychiatry. 1977;**40**:1072-1082. DOI: 10.1136/jnnp.40.11.1072

[56] Pham M, Oikonomou D, Hornung B, Weiler M, Heiland S, Bäumer P, et al. Magnetic resonance neurography detects diabetic neuropathy early and with proximal predominance. Annals of Neurology. 2015;**78**:939-948. DOI: 10.1002/ana.24524

[57] Dyck PJ, Lais A, Karnes JL, O'Brien P, Rizza R. Fiber loss is primary and multifocal in sural nerves in diabetic polyneuropathy. Annals of Neurology. 1986;**19**:425-439. DOI: 10.1002/ana.410190503

[58] Kobayashi M, Zochodne DW. Diabetic neuropathy and the sensory neuron: New aspects of pathogenesis and their treatment implications. Journal of Diabetes Investigation. 2018;**9**:1239-1254. DOI: 10.1111/jdi.12833

[59] Jende JME, Kender Z, Mooshage C, Groener JB, Alvarez-Ramos L, Kollmer J, et al. Diffusion tensor imaging of the sciatic nerve as a surrogate marker for nerve functionality of the upper and lower limb in patients with diabetes and prediabetes. Frontiers in Neuroscience. 2021;**15**:642589. DOI: 10.3389/fnins.2021.642589

[60] Planté-Bordeneuve V, Said G. Familial amyloid polyneuropathy. Lancet Neurology. 2011;**10**:1086-1097. DOI: 10.1016/S1474-4422(11)70246-0

[61] Kollmer J, Hegenbart U, Kimmich C, Hund E, Purrucker JC, Hayes JM, et al. Magnetization transfer ratio quantifies polyneuropathy in hereditary transthyretin amyloidosis. Annals of Clinical Translational Neurology. 2020;**7**:799-807. DOI: 10.1002/acn3.51049

[62] Adams D, Gonzalez-Duarte A, O'Riordan WD, Yang C-C, Ueda M, Kristen AV, et al. Patisiran, an RNAi therapeutic, for hereditary transthyretin amyloidosis. The New England Journal of Medicine. 2018;**379**:11-21. DOI: 10.1056/NEJMoa1716153

[63] Coelho T, Maia LF, Martins da Silva A, Waddington Cruz M, Planté-Bordeneuve V, Lozeron P, et al. Tafamidis for transthyretin familial amyloid polyneuropathy: A randomized, controlled trial. Neurology. 2012;**79**:785-792. DOI: 10.1212/WNL.0b013e3182661eb1

[64] Shahrizaila N, Lehmann HC, Kuwabara S. Guillain-Barré syndrome. The Lancet. 2021;**397**:1214-1228. DOI: 10.1016/S0140-6736(21)00517-1

[65] Grimm A, Oertl H, Auffenberg E, Schubert V, Ruschil C, Axer H, et al. Differentiation between Guillain–Barré syndrome and acute-onset chronic inflammatory demyelinating polyradiculoneuritis—A prospective follow-up study using ultrasound and neurophysiological measurements. Neurotherapeutics. 2019;**16**:838-847. DOI: 10.1007/s13311-019-00716-5

[66] Abreu E, Aubert S, Wavreille G, Gheno R, Canella C, Cotten A. Peripheral tumor and tumor-like neurogenic lesions. European Journal of Radiology. 2013;**82**:38-50. DOI: 10.1016/j.ejrad.2011.04.036

[67] Ahlawat S, Fayad LM, Khan MS, Bredella MA, Harris GJ, Evans DG, et al.

Current whole-body MRI applications in the neurofibromatoses: NF1, NF2, and schwannomatosis. Neurology. 2016;**87**:S31-S39. DOI: 10.1212/WNL.0000000000002929

[68] Liebig. Perineural invasion in cancer. Cancer. 2009. DOI: 10.1002/cncr.24396 [Accessed: February 18, 2025]

[69] Crush AB, Howe BM, Spinner RJ, Amrami KK, Hunt CH, Johnson GB, et al. Malignant involvement of the peripheral nervous system in patients with cancer: Multimodality imaging and pathologic correlation. Radiographics. 2014;**34**:1987-2007. DOI: 10.1148/rg.347130129

[70] Martinoli C, Derchi LE, Bertolotto M, Gandolfo N, Bianchi S, Fiallo P, et al. US and MR imaging of peripheral nerves in leprosy. Skeletal Radiology. 2000;**29**:142-150. DOI: 10.1007/s002560050584

[71] Upadhyaya V, Upadhyaya DN, Bansal R, Pandey T, Pandey AK. MR neurography in parsonage-turner syndrome. Indian Journal Of Radiology And Imaging. 2021;**29**:264-270. DOI: 10.4103/ijri.IJRI_269_19

[72] Wadhwa V, Scott KM, Rozen S, Starr AJ, Chhabra A. CT-guided perineural injections for chronic pelvic pain. RadioGraphics. 2016;**36**:1408-1425. DOI: 10.1148/rg.2016150263

[73] Michaud K, Cooper P, Abd-Elsayed A, Kohan L. Review of radiofrequency ablation for peripheral nerves. Current Pain and Headache Reports. 2021;**25**(10). DOI: 10.1007/s11916-021-00981-0

[74] Naskar S, Bhoi D, Hoda W, Garg H. Cryoablation in chronic pain management: A narrative review. Indian Journal of Pain. 2024;**38**:161. DOI: 10.4103/ijpn.ijpn_47_24

[75] Rojo-Manaute JM, Capa-Grasa A, Chana-Rodríguez F, Perez-Mañanes R, Rodriguez-Maruri G, Sanz-Ruiz P, et al. Ultra-minimally invasive ultrasound-guided carpal tunnel release: A randomized clinical trial. Journal of Ultrasound in Medicine Off J Am Inst Ultrasound Med. 2016;**35**:1149-1157. DOI: 10.7863/ultra.15.07001

[76] Chou RC, Robinson DM, Homer S. Ultrasound-guided percutaneous carpal tunnel release: A systematic review. PM&R. 2023;**15**:363-379. DOI: 10.1002/pmrj.12801

[77] Qin J, Wang L, Sun Y, Sun X, Wen C, Shahmoradi M, et al. Concentrated growth factor increases Schwann cell proliferation and neurotrophic factor secretion and promotes functional nerve recovery in vivo. International Journal of Molecular Medicine. 2016;**37**:493-500. DOI: 10.3892/ijmm.2015.2438

[78] Catapano M, Catapano J, Borschel G, Alavinia SM, Robinson LR, Mittal N. Effectiveness of platelet-rich plasma injections for nonsurgical management of carpal tunnel syndrome: A systematic review and meta-analysis of randomized controlled trials. Archives of Physical Medicine and Rehabilitation. 2020;**101**:897-906. DOI: 10.1016/j.apmr.2019.10.193

[79] Wang S, Liu X, Wang Y. Evaluation of platelet-rich plasma therapy for peripheral nerve regeneration: A critical review of literature. 2022;**10**. DOI: 10.3389/fbioe.2022.808248

Section 3

Metabolic Neuropathies and Clinical Guidelines

Chapter 3

Treatment Options for Diabetic Neuropathy: Insights from the Romanian Neuropathy Guidelines

Andra-Elena Nica, Oana Andreea Parliteanu, Sivu Claudia, Carmen Dobjanschi, Emilia Rusu and Gabriela Radulian

Abstract

Diabetic neuropathy is a common and debilitating complication of diabetes mellitus, requiring a multidisciplinary approach for effective management. It encompasses a broad spectrum of neurological impairments, including sensory, motor, and autonomic dysfunctions, significantly impacting patients' quality of life and increasing morbidity. Despite advances in diabetes care, its global prevalence continues to rise, contributing to a substantial healthcare burden. The pathophysiology is multifactorial, involving oxidative stress, mitochondrial dysfunction, chronic hyperglycemia, and neuroinflammation, leading to progressive neuronal degeneration. Early diagnosis is critical, as nerve dysfunction may begin in the prediabetic stage. Diagnostic evaluation includes clinical assessment, electrophysiological testing, and emerging modalities such as corneal confocal microscopy and sudomotor function testing. The clinical presentation varies, with distal symmetric polyneuropathy being the most prevalent form, followed by autonomic neuropathy, which affects cardiovascular, gastrointestinal, and genitourinary systems, leading to severe complications. Prevention remains the primary strategy, emphasizing optimal glycemic control, lifestyle modifications, and risk factor management. Pharmacologic treatment is aimed at symptomatic relief and neuroprotection, utilizing agents such as pregabalin, duloxetine, and alpha-lipoic acid. Emerging therapeutic approaches, including neuromodulation and regenerative therapies, hold promise for improved patient outcomes. Comprehensive multidisciplinary care, patient education, and individualized treatment strategies are essential to prevent complications such as foot ulcers, infections, and amputations. Further research is needed to explore novel therapeutic targets and optimize current management strategies for diabetic neuropathy.

Keywords: diabetic neuropathy, treatment, guidelines, pain management, nerve protection, Romanian neuropathy guidelines

IntechOpen

1. Introduction

The management of individuals with diabetes mellitus (DM) and its chronic complications requires a comprehensive, multidisciplinary approach that extends beyond the boundaries of distinct medical specialties.

Diabetic neuropathy is defined by anatomical, clinical, neurological, and metabolic disturbances occurring in the course of DM, after excluding other potential etiologies such as hereditary, traumatic, neoplastic, infectious, compressive, metabolic, or autoimmune causes.

Despite advancements in diabetes care, polyneuropathy remains a highly prevalent complication, with a lifetime prevalence exceeding 50% [1]. As the disease progresses, approximately half of the individuals with diabetes will develop DPN making it the primary cause for foot ulcers as well as disability and amputation rates [2]. By 2045, it is estimated that 783 million adults worldwide will have diabetes, of whom 350 million will develop diabetic polyneuropathy. This complication is associated with significant morbidity, including an increased risk of trauma (patients with peripheral neuropathy have a 2–3 times higher risk of falls), ulceration (15% of affected individuals will develop an ulcer at some point), infections, and an up to 15-fold increased risk of amputations [3].

Diabetic neuropathy significantly impairs quality of life, leading to chronic pain, sleep disturbances, and reduced mobility. Studies indicate that up to 80% of patients experience depression or anxiety related to neuropathic pain [4, 5]. The persistent nature of pain, along with associated motor and sensory deficits, contributes to reduced independence in daily activities, increased risk of falls, and diminished social interactions. Sleep disorders, including insomnia and restless leg syndrome, are commonly reported in patients with neuropathy, further exacerbating fatigue and psychological distress.

Validated assessment tools such as the Michigan Neuropathy Screening Instrument (MNSI) and the Neuropathy Disability Score (NDS) should be routinely used to monitor disease progression and treatment response. Additionally, patient-reported outcome measures (PROMs) such as the Brief Pain Inventory (BPI) and the Diabetic Neuropathy Symptom Score (DNSS) can provide valuable insights into the real-world impact of the condition on patients' well-being. Addressing neuropathy-related impairments through multidisciplinary pain management, psychological support, and rehabilitative therapies is essential to enhancing quality of life in affected individuals.

The prevalence of peripheral neuropathy in the prediabetic stage is estimated to be as high as 18%, suggesting that neuronal alterations occur early in glycemic imbalance, particularly affecting small fibers. It is estimated that 20 years after the onset of type 1 DM, approximately 30% of patients develop cardiovascular autonomic neuropathy, whereas in type 2 DM, this prevalence increases to 60% after 15 years of disease progression [3].

2. Diabetic neuropathy

2.1 Etiology and pathogenesis

The pathogenesis of peripheral neuropathy is multifactorial and includes oxidative stress [6], mitochondrial dysfunction, inflammatory changes, advanced glycation

DOI: http://dx.doi.org/10.5772/intechopen.1009813

end-product formation, polyol pathway activation, and reduced oxygen and glucose availability for neuronal cells due to localized microangiopathy at the vasa nervorum [3, 7]. Neuronal dysfunction results from alterations in the blood-nerve barrier, leading to increased permeability, neuroinflammation, endoneurial hypoxia, and pericyte dysfunction. Increased permeability of this barrier causes the accumulation of proteins (albumin, IgG, IgM, and mannitol) in the endoneurium, disrupting osmotic balance and resulting in edema. Metabolic disturbances, such as chronic hyperglycemia and excessive free fatty acids, may contribute to blood-nerve barrier damage through direct toxicity. Local nerve inflammation triggers cytokine and chemokine secretion by Schwann cells, leading to leukocyte extravasation [7, 8]. This inflammatory response, combined with increased membrane permeability, contributes to progressive neuronal degeneration, which cannot be counteracted by anti-inflammatory macrophages, thereby promoting chronic inflammation. Neuropathy, in turn, induces the opening of vascular shunts, causing capillary bypassing of blood flow, further exacerbating ischemia [9].

Risk factors for neuropathy development include advanced age, duration of diabetes or glycemic imbalance (prediabetes), poor glycemic control, and frequent episodes of hypoglycemia (which reduce intraneuronal metabolite concentrations, leading to axonal degeneration and Schwann cell myelin degradation), as well as local ischemia [7]. Additional risk factors may include hypertension, dyslipidemia, chronic smoking, and obesity [2, 4, 10]. While some of these factors are non-modifiable, most can be addressed through lifestyle modifications and appropriate pharmacologic interventions, thereby preventing or slowing the progression of neuropathy.

2.2 Classification

1. *Distal Symmetric Sensorimotor Polyneuropathy* – The most common type of diabetic neuropathy (75% of cases), characterized by peripheral sensory loss (thermal, proprioceptive, pain, and tactile), followed by motor impairment [5].

    - *Small fiber neuropathy* – An early manifestation of diabetic neuropathy (sometimes occurring as early as the prediabetes stage), challenging to diagnose as sensory testing may yield normal results. It is frequently associated with altered pain and thermal sensitivity [2, 3].

    - *Large fiber neuropathy* – Characterized by loss of proprioceptive and vibratory sensation and sensory ataxia [3].

    - *Mixed neuropathy* – Involves both large and small fiber impairment.

2. *Diabetic Autonomic Neuropathy* – A widespread condition affecting cholinergic, adrenergic, and peptidergic fibers in the context of diabetes mellitus (in the absence of other causes):

    - Cardiovascular involvement

    - Gastrointestinal involvement

    - Genitourinary dysfunction

- Sudomotor dysfunction
- Ocular involvement

3. *Proximal motor neuropathy – radiculoplexopathy (diabetic amyotrophy)* – Primarily affects the lumbosacral plexus but may also involve the cervical plexus. Histopathological examination suggests ischemia and microvasculitis [2].

4. *Multiple mononeuropathy* – Occurs in the absence of rheumatologic disease [2]; affects one or more contiguous nerve roots and is associated with advanced age (over 50 years) and male sex.

5. *Mononeuropathies:*

   - *Cranial mononeuropathy* – Most commonly affects the oculomotor nerve (III), followed by the trochlear (IV) and facial (VII) nerves. Oculomotor nerve palsy with pupillary sparing is a characteristic sign of diabetic cranial nerve III involvement due to vascular compromise and nerve infarction.

   - *Peripheral mononeuropathy* – Most frequently involves the median, ulnar, radial, common peroneal, and lateral femoral cutaneous nerves.

6. *Polyradiculoneuropathies* – Occur in the absence of compressive causes.

7. *Medication-induced neuropathy* – Presents as acute pain and/or autonomic dysfunction following the initiation of insulin therapy, caused by a rapid decline in blood glucose levels or an overly aggressive improvement in glycemic control (a decrease of more than 2% in HbA1c within 3 months). Symptoms may include severe, treatment-resistant pain, autonomic dysfunction, worsening nephropathy, or retinopathy. The underlying cause is endoneurial edema and ischemia [2, 3].

2.3 Clinical manifestations

1. *Distal symmetric sensorimotor polyneuropathy* – The typical presentation follows a "glove" or "stocking" distribution, with burning pain, dysesthesia (when small fibers are affected), paresthesia, tingling, pain upon touch, muscle cramps, restless legs, muscle weakness, gait instability, and Charcot foot (when large fibers are involved) [3, 5].

   - Sensory manifestations typically precede motor symptoms and are more frequently observed. Patients often describe the paradox of experiencing numbness in their lower limbs while simultaneously having heightened sensitivity, to the extent that they cannot tolerate contact with socks or bed sheets. Neuropathic pain is characterized by burning and stabbing sensations, often associated with allodynia and hypnalgia (pain exacerbation in the evening or at night) [2, 3].

2. *Autonomic neuropathy:*

   - *Cardiovascular autonomic neuropathy (CAN):* Often overlooked in clinical practice, CAN has serious health consequences. It is a major cause of morbidity and mortality in patients with diabetes, serving as an independent risk factor for cardiac arrhythmias, silent myocardial ischemia, and sudden cardiac death. CAN is influenced by multiple factors, including diabetes duration, chronic hyperglycemia severity, coexisting atherosclerotic coronary disease, hypertension, and hypercholesterolemia. Clinical symptoms typically manifest in advanced stages as exercise intolerance, resting tachycardia, and orthostatic hypotension, which is defined as a drop in systolic blood pressure by >20 mmHg and/or diastolic blood pressure by >10 mmHg upon standing [11].

Subclinical CAN is characterized by reduced heart rate variability and abnormal cardiovascular reflex testing. It can be detected as early as 1 year after a type 2 diabetes diagnosis and 5 years after type 1 diabetes diagnosis [12].

- *Gastrointestinal autonomic neuropathy:* This can affect any part of the gastrointestinal tract, manifesting as esophageal dysmotility, gastroparesis, constipation, diarrhea, and fecal incontinence. Associated symptoms include nausea, vomiting, bloating, early satiety, alternating constipation and diarrhea, delayed gastric emptying, and gastroesophageal reflux.

Gastroparesis should be suspected in individuals with poorly controlled diabetes or unexplained upper gastrointestinal symptoms [3].

- *Genitourinary autonomic neuropathy:* Leads to sexual and bladder dysfunction. In men, diabetic autonomic neuropathy can cause erectile dysfunction and/or retrograde ejaculation [3]. Due to its association with endothelial dysfunction, erectile dysfunction serves as an early marker of cardiovascular disease. In women, sexual dysfunction is more common in those with diabetes and is characterized by reduced sexual desire, dyspareunia, diminished arousal, and inadequate lubrication [13].

- Neurogenic bladder dysfunction presents with difficulty initiating urination, prolonged voiding intervals, post-micturition dribbling, nocturnal incontinence, and, in severe cases, acute urinary retention. Due to bladder atony and increased post-void residual volumes, urinary tract infections are common.

- *Diabetic cystopathy* results from sacral nerve involvement, and while some patients remain asymptomatic, others experience urinary incontinence, partial or complete urinary retention, nocturia, polyuria, and urgency.

- *Sudomotor dysfunction:* Thermoregulatory disturbances involve reduced or absent sweating in some areas and excessive sweating after food ingestion. The most common manifestations include the following:

- *Distal anhidrosis:* Symmetric absence of sweating on the soles, with a tendency to spread proximally. It may be associated with compensatory hyperhidrosis in the upper body (often mistaken for hypoglycemic episodes).

- *Heat intolerance:* Patients report an increased sensitivity to heat rather than noticing hypohidrosis. Sweating abnormalities result from sympathetic denervation of sweat glands, with lesions located in peripheral nerve fibers.

- *Gustatory sweating:* Profuse sweating on the face and hands during meals, likely due to aberrant autonomic innervation.

- *Distal anhidrosis*, characterized by the absence of sweating on the soles, is bilaterally symmetric with a progressive extension. It may be associated with compensatory hyperhidrosis in the upper body, which is often mistaken for signs of a hypoglycemic episode.

- *Heat intolerance*, where patients report increased sensitivity to heat but may be less aware of hypohidrosis. Sudomotor dysfunction results from sympathetic denervation of sweat glands, with lesions primarily affecting peripheral nerve fibers.

- *Gustatory sweating*, which presents as excessive sweating on the face and hands during meals, likely due to aberrant autonomic innervation.

- *Ocular involvement*: Patients may exhibit miosis with delayed adaptation to darkness and impaired night vision.

3. *Radiculoplexopathy*: Patients present with weight loss, pain, and muscle weakness in the distribution of one or more thoracic or lumbar nerves. The most common form is *diabetic amyotrophy*, which begins with acute, asymmetric pain localized to one lower limb, followed by progressive muscle weakness in the affected leg. The condition evolves over several months, with partial recovery and possible residual neuropathic pain. The contralateral limb may also become involved within days or later in the disease course [2]. In cases of cervical radiculoplexopathy, increasing pain intensity necessitates the exclusion of spinal cord compression.

4. *Mononeuropathies*:

- *Cranial nerve III*: Characterized by unilateral pain, ptosis, and diplopia, with preservation of pupillary function, which is a hallmark of diabetic oculomotor nerve palsy due to vascular infarction [2].

- *Ulnar nerve*: Presents with paresthesia and sensory deficits in the fifth digit and medial half of the fourth digit, along with motor impairment affecting the intrinsic hand muscles. Severe cases result in a "claw hand" deformity due to muscle atrophy.

- *Radial nerve*: Manifests as wrist drop (motor deficit in wrist extensors) and sensory disturbances in the first interosseous space.

- *Peroneal nerve*: Presents with foot drop due to motor impairment of the foot extensors.

- *Lateral femoral cutaneous nerve*: Causes sensory deficits in the anterolateral thigh.

2.4 Diagnosis

Peripheral neuropathy screening should begin at the time of type 2 diabetes (T2DM) diagnosis and 5 years after the onset of type 1 diabetes (T1DM), with annual follow-ups thereafter, as per clinical guidelines [3].

Since studies have shown that neuropathic changes can start in the prediabetes stage, screening may be performed from the moment of prediabetes diagnosis [14].

The diagnosis of peripheral neuropathy involves multiple steps:

a. *Comprehensive history* (detailed anamnesis).

b. *Bilateral sensory examination*, including:

- Pain perception (pinprick).
- Vibration sense (128 Hz tuning fork).
- Pressure sensation (10 g monofilament).
- Thermal sensation (thermotest) [15, 16].

c. *Electromyography (EMG)* – Measures nerve conduction velocity in skeletal muscles (commonly peroneal, tibial, ulnar, median, and sural nerves) using needle electrodes that record resting and contraction-induced potentials. Pathological changes may include spontaneous fibrillation potentials at rest, decreased nerve conduction velocity, and reduced response amplitude [17].

d. *Nerve biopsy* – Reserved for cases where neuropathy etiology is difficult to determine.

e. *Emerging diagnostic methods:*

- *Small fiber neuropathy tests:*
    - *Neuropad* (plantar patch measuring sudomotor function; sensitivity 86%, specificity 65%) [18, 19].
    - *Sudoscan* test evaluates autonomic nerve function by measuring sweat gland response to stimuli. It provides important insights into early neuropathic changes, particularly in small fiber neuropathy. While its sensitivity is well-documented, challenges related to equipment availability and standardization of testing protocols have hindered widespread adoption. Further research is needed to establish its role in routine clinical assessment and improve accessibility.
    - *Skin biopsy* (gold standard for evaluating intraepidermal nerve fiber density).
    - *Corneal confocal microscopy* (assesses small nerve fiber loss in the cornea and correlates with somatic neuropathy severity and progression) [18]. It has demonstrated high sensitivity in detecting small fiber neuropathy and correlates well with traditional measures of nerve dysfunction. Its use is limited by high costs and the need for specialized equipment, making it less accessible in routine clinical practice. Despite these barriers, it remains a valuable tool for early neuropathy detection and monitoring disease progression.

- *Large fiber neuropathy tests:*
  - o *Automated NCS* (measures sural nerve conduction velocity and response amplitude; sensitivity 90.48%, specificity 86.11%) [20, 21].
  - o *VibraTip™* (a small device producing vibrations similar to a 128 Hz tuning fork; sensitivity 95%, specificity 95%) [22].
- *Clinical scales and questionnaires:*
  - o *Michigan Neuropathy Screening Instrument (MNSI):* A 15-question survey combined with sensory testing, reflex assessment, and foot inspection. A score > 7 is considered abnormal [7].
  - o *Toronto Clinical Scoring System (CSS):* Evaluates symptoms, Achilles and patellar reflexes, and sensory testing, with a score range from 0 to 19.
  - o *Neuropathy Symptom Score (NSS):* Assesses symptom severity based on 17 questions.
  - o *Neuropathy Disability Score (NDS):* Evaluates neuropathic impairment through vibration, thermal, pressure sensation testing, and Achilles reflex assessment. Neuropathy is classified as absent, mild, moderate, or severe based on the total score.
  - o *Leeds Assessment of Neuropathic Symptoms and Signs (LANSS) Pain Scale:* Differentiates neuropathic pain from other pain types, incorporating five symptoms and two clinical signs of distal polyneuropathy.
  - o *NeuroQol:* Assesses quality of life in neuropathy patients.
  - o *Utah Early Neuropathy Scale (UENS):* Detects early small fiber neuropathy by evaluating pain sensitivity, allodynia, hyperesthesia, tendon reflexes, and motor deficits, with a maximum score of 42 [18, 23].

For patients with diabetic neuropathy and diabetes mellitus, other potential neuropathy etiologies must be considered, including toxins (e.g., alcohol use), neurotoxic medications (e.g., chemotherapeutic agents), vitamin B12 deficiency, hypothyroidism, renal disease, malignancies (e.g., multiple myeloma), chronic infections (e.g., HIV), chronic inflammatory demyelinating polyneuropathy, hereditary neuropathies, and vasculitis [24].

Emerging diagnostic modalities such as corneal confocal microscopy and sudomotor function testing have demonstrated high sensitivity for detecting small fiber neuropathy. Their integration into routine clinical practice is limited by high costs and restricted availability in many regions. Automated nerve conduction studies (NCS) and novel skin biopsy techniques provide additional diagnostic value, but further efforts are needed to improve their accessibility.

2.5 Diagnosis of autonomic neuropathies

Screening is recommended for patients with type 1 diabetes (T1DM) after 5 years of disease progression and annually for those with type 2 diabetes (T2DM) [24].

- *Cardiovascular autonomic neuropathy (CAN):* Several diagnostic approaches, varying in complexity, are used in clinical practice and research. These include cardiovascular reflex testing, heart rate variability analysis, orthostatic hypotension assessment, ECG with QT interval measurement, 24-hour blood pressure monitoring, baroreflex sensitivity testing, cardiac scintigraphy, microneurography, and venous occlusion plethysmography [11].

  Based on existing evidence, the Toronto Diabetic Neuropathy Consensus Meeting concluded that cardiovascular reflex testing is a sensitive, specific, reproducible, safe, and standardized method. It was recommended as the reference standard for clinical assessment of autonomic function [25–28]. In advanced CAN, resting tachycardia (>100 bpm) and orthostatic hypotension (a repeated drop in systolic blood pressure by >20 mmHg or diastolic blood pressure by >10 mmHg upon standing) are frequently observed [11, 24].

- *Gastrointestinal autonomic neuropathy:* Before considering a diagnosis or specialized testing for gastroparesis, organic causes of gastric outlet obstruction or peptic ulcer disease must be ruled out through esophagogastroduodenoscopy or barium swallow studies. The gold standard for gastroparesis diagnosis is *gastric emptying scintigraphy*, measuring solid food retention at 15-minute intervals over 4 hours. The *13C-octanoic acid breath test* is a viable alternative [29].

- *Genitourinary autonomic neuropathy:* Bladder function assessment should be performed in diabetic patients with a history of recurrent urinary tract infections, pyelonephritis, incontinence, or bladder distention.

- *Ocular autonomic dysfunction:* Clinically manifests as delayed pupillary response to light adaptation, leading to impaired night vision.

2.6 Management

Prevention is the most crucial strategy in the management of neuropathy, focusing on optimal metabolic control from the prediabetes stage to prevent irreversible neuronal damage. Maintaining adequate metabolic control delays the onset of neuropathy and slows its progression [10].

Strict glycemic control reduces the relative risk of neuropathy by *78% in type 1 diabetes and 5–9% in type 2 diabetes* [3]. The difference arises from multiple comorbidities associated with type 2 diabetes, differences in treatment regimens, frequency of hypoglycemic episodes, age, and weight status between type 1 and type 2 diabetes patients. Lifestyle modifications, including *physical activity, weight loss, and dietary changes*, have demonstrated benefits in slowing neuropathy progression, reducing symptom severity, and even promoting nerve fiber regeneration.

The *BARDI 2D study* (Bypass Angioplasty Revascularization Investigation in Type 2 Diabetes) found a lower incidence of distal diabetic neuropathy at 4 years in patients treated with insulin-sensitizing agents compared to those receiving insulin/sulfonylurea therapy. Additionally, the *ACCORD trial* (Action to Control Cardiovascular Risk in Diabetes) showed significant benefits of intensive glycemic and blood pressure management in preventing diabetic autonomic neuropathy in type 2 diabetes [30].

3. Lipid and blood pressure control

- *Dyslipidemia* is a major risk factor for diabetic neuropathy in type 2 diabetes and may also contribute to neuropathy risk in type 1 diabetes [30–32]. However, no clear benefit has been demonstrated for using statins or other lipid-lowering agents in preventing diabetic polyneuropathy.

- *Hypertension:* A recent meta-analysis of patients from 14 countries (*INTERPRET-DD study*) identified hypertension as an independent risk factor for diabetic peripheral polyneuropathy (odds ratio 1.58) [33]. The *ACCORD trial* found that intensive blood pressure management reduced the risk of *cardiac autonomic neuropathy by 25%* [34].

3.1 Treatment of peripheral neuropathy

3.1.1 Non-pharmacological treatment

- Transcutaneous electrical nerve stimulation (TENS)

- Frequency-modulated electromagnetic nerve stimulation (FREMS)

- High-tone external muscle stimulation therapy

- Acupuncture

- Psychological support

These approaches provide *modest pain relief* and may serve as adjunctive therapies alongside pharmacologic treatment.

3.1.2 Pharmacologic treatment

- *Pathogenic treatment*:

  o *Alpha-lipoic acid* – A potent antioxidant administered orally or intravenously.

  o *Benfotiamine* – A synthetic vitamin B1 derivative that is absorbed as thiamine; it reduces the accumulation of pyruvate, lactate, and alpha-ketoglutarate in blood and tissues.

- *Symptomatic treatment*: First-line pharmacologic agents for neuropathic pain include *duloxetine, pregabalin, and gabapentin* [2, 3, 35].

  o *Pregabalin* – A calcium channel modulator that inhibits neurotransmitter release; studies show it reduces pain by *30–50%* [2, 3, 35].

  o *Duloxetine* – A *selective serotonin and norepinephrine reuptake inhibitor (SNRI)*, shown to be more effective than pregabalin for pain reduction; both medications have *good tolerability and mild side effects* (loss of appetite, drowsiness, nausea, vomiting, constipation, orthostatic hypotension) [2, 3, 35].

- o *Gabapentin* – A calcium channel ligand similar to pregabalin; requires dose titration, with *age-dependent variations in side effect severity* (**Table 1**) [2, 3, 35].

3.1.3 Second-line pharmacologic treatment for neuropathic pain

A. *Tricyclic antidepressants (TCAs):* Amitriptyline, nortriptyline, venlafaxine, and desvenlafaxine are considered second-line treatment options. Most act as serotonin-norepinephrine reuptake inhibitors. Although they reduce neuropathic pain symptoms, they have multiple dose-dependent adverse effects, primarily due to *antimuscarinic properties* (xerostomia, constipation, blurred vision, urinary retention, nausea, vomiting, hypotension, vertigo) [2, 3].

- *Amitriptyline* is the most commonly used TCA: the dose is gradually increased, starting from *25 mg/day*, up to *150 mg/day*, if necessary. The *maintenance dose* is typically *50–100 mg/day*. In elderly patients, dose escalation should be done progressively under medical supervision.

B. *Opioids (tapentadol and tramadol):* These drugs act as *opioid receptor agonists* and inhibit norepinephrine reuptake. Their use in neuropathic pain is controversial due to *limited efficacy* compared to the *high risk of dependence*. They should only be considered *after all other treatment options have been exhausted* [2, 3].

- *Tapentadol:* Initial dose *50 mg (single dose)*; doses above *600 mg/day* have not been studied and are therefore *not recommended*. If discontinuation is required, the dose should be tapered gradually to avoid withdrawal symptoms.
  - o *Adverse effects:* Dependence (!), dizziness, drowsiness, headache, nausea, constipation, decreased appetite, attention deficit, dyspnea.
- *Tramadol:* Recommended dose is *50 mg;* if ineffective, another dose may be given within *30–60 minutes*. The *maximum daily dose should not exceed 400 mg*.
  - o *Adverse effects:* Dependence (!), vertigo, visual disturbances, palpitations, tachycardia, dyspnea, nausea, excessive sweating.

C. *Other treatment options:*

- *Novel analgesics – Lacosamide* [36] and *Mirogabalin* (a gabapentinoid acting on voltage-dependent calcium channels, with a *longer duration of action* and *greater potency* than gabapentin) [37].

Drug	Dosage	Mechanism of action	Efficacy	Safety profile	Cost-effectiveness
Pregabalin	150–600 mg/day	Calcium channel modulator	Moderate-high	Dizziness, weight gain	Moderate
Duloxetine	60–120 mg/day	SNRI	High	Nausea, dry mouth	High
Gabapentin	300–3600 mg/day	Calcium channel modulator	Moderate	Sedation, dizziness	Low

Table 1.
First-line symptomatic pharmacologic treatment for peripheral neuropathy.

Drug	Initial dose	Maximum dose	Adverse effects
Lacosamide	100–200 mg/day	600 mg/day	Dizziness, headache, nausea, tinnitus, depression, confusion, insomnia, tremor, nystagmus, and dysarthria
Capsaicin patch	1 patch, applied for 30 minutes	4 patches	Burning sensation, ocular irritation, first-degree atrioventricular block, hypertension, cough, nausea, pruritus, pain, and erythema at the application site

Table 2.
Additional analgesic options for peripheral neuropathy.

- *Clonidine gel* – found to be *non-inferior to capsaicin*, with *fewer adverse effects* [38].
- *Capsaicin patch* – used for localized pain relief [2, 38].
- *Lidocaine patch* – offers *fewer side effects* than systemic treatment [2, 38].
- *Anti-NGF (nerve growth factor) antibodies – Tanezumab (subcutaneous administration), Fulranumab* [39].
- *Cannabinoid inhalations – Dose-dependent effects*, possible *euphoric effect* [38].
- *Sodium channel blockers – Lamotrigine, lacosamide, carbamazepine, oxcarbazepine, valproic acid* [40].

D. *Capsaicin:* a *capsaicinoid extract* from chili peppers, used as a topical analgesic in *diabetic neuropathy, postherpetic neuralgia, and HIV-associated neuropathy*. It depolarizes neuronal membranes, producing a sensation similar to *intense heat or burning* (**Table 2**) [2].

3.1.4 Additional pathogenic treatment options

Other agents targeting pathogenic mechanisms include:

- *Metanx* (combination of L-methylfolate, methylcobalamin, and pyridoxal-5-phosphate), with *good tolerability* [41].
- *ARA 290* (an erythropoietin analog), effective in *improving paresthesia, thermal sensitivity, and allodynia* [42].
- *Actovegin*, which enhances *oxygen and glucose utilization at the neuronal level*; effects appear after prolonged use, with *no reported adverse effects* [38].

4. Non-pharmacologic and emerging therapies

- Non-pharmacologic interventions are gaining recognition as essential components of neuropathy management. *Neuromodulation techniques, including spinal cord stimulation and transcutaneous electrical nerve stimulation* (TENS), have shown promise in reducing pain and improving nerve function. TENS therapy is particularly useful in modulating pain perception through peripheral nerve stimulation, offering an alternative for patients who are intolerant to pharmacological agents. Spinal cord stimulation, though more invasive, has demonstrated efficacy in refractory neuropathic pain cases.

- *Regenerative medicine approaches*, such as *stem cell therapy and nerve growth factor administration*, are currently being explored as potential disease-modifying treatments. Stem cell therapy aims to restore nerve function by promoting axonal regeneration and reducing inflammation. Experimental studies have shown that mesenchymal stem cells can enhance neuronal repair mechanisms, but clinical implementation is still in early phases. Nerve growth factors, including brain-derived neurotrophic factor (BDNF) and vascular endothelial growth factor (VEGF), have shown promise in stimulating nerve regeneration, though their therapeutic application remains under investigation.

4.1 Autonomic neuropathy treatment

4.1.1 Management of cardiovascular autonomic neuropathy (CAN)

An *effective preventive strategy* for CAN should include the following:

- Weight management
- Physical activity
- Smoking cessation
- Nutritional planning
- Metabolic optimization
- Cardiovascular risk factor control (e.g., hypertension and dyslipidemia)
- Behavioral approaches to stress management [43].

The *Toronto Consensus* concluded that *lifestyle optimization interventions can improve heart rate variability in diabetes and prediabetes*. The *ADA (American Diabetes Association)* recommends *lifestyle modification* as a strategy to improve CAN in diabetic patients [44].

There is *strong evidence* supporting *intensive hyperglycemia management in type 1 diabetes* (proven by the *EDIC study*) [45], while in *type 2 diabetes*, effective CAN prevention is only evident in the *context of a multifactorial management strategy* [46]. The ADA *recommends early glycemic control optimization to prevent or delay CAN in type 1 diabetes* and a *multifactorial approach* targeting both *glycemia and cardiovascular risk factors* for CAN prevention in type 2 diabetes [3].

4.1.2 Management of orthostatic hypotension

Treatment is *only recommended for symptomatic cases*, aiming to *minimize symptoms and improve quality of life. Non-pharmacological measures* are often sufficient and should be prioritized.

- *First step: exclude or reduce medications* that may worsen orthostatic hypotension.
- *Supportive interventions: light physical exercises and rapid intake of 500 mL of water* are recommended [47].
- *Additional non-pharmacological measures:*

  o *Compression stockings (worn over calves and abdomen)*

  o *Adequate salt intake* [48].

4.1.3 Pharmacologic treatment of orthostatic hypotension

Patient education is *an essential element* of the management strategy. Treating hypertension in these patients can be challenging due to *the need to lower blood pressure without exacerbating orthostatic hypotension*.

Recommended pharmacologic options:

- *Short-acting agents that also influence baroreceptor activity*, such as *guanabenz or clonidine*.
- *Short-acting calcium channel blockers*, such as *isradipine*.

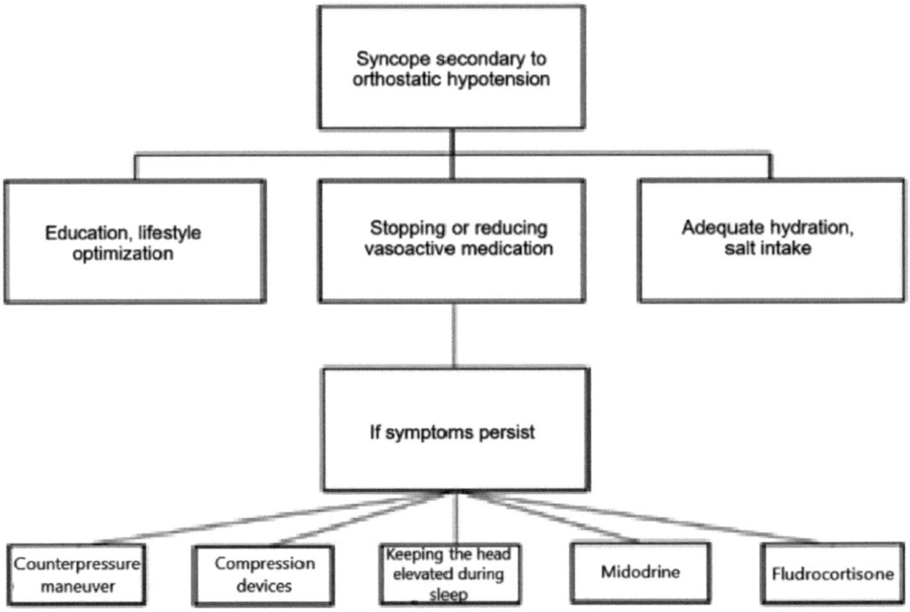

Figure 1.
Non-pharmacological treatment for orthostatic hypotension.

- *Short-acting beta-blockers*, such as *atenolol or metoprolol tartrate*.

- *Enalapril* as an alternative for patients intolerant to the above medications [49–51].

- *Midodrine (2.5–10 mg/day)* and *droxidopa (100–600 mg/day)* are *FDA-approved* for the treatment of *orthostatic hypotension* (**Figure 1**).

5. Treatment of gastroparesis

Managing diabetic gastroparesis can be challenging [52]. Dietary recommendations include a low-fiber, low-fat meal plan, with small, frequent meals and a higher proportion of calories derived from liquid foods [53–55].

Discontinuing medications that negatively affect gastrointestinal motility, such as opioids, anticholinergics, tricyclic antidepressants, GLP-1 receptor agonists, pramlintide, and possibly DPP-4 inhibitors, may also improve gastric motility [53, 54].

In severe cases, pharmacological intervention is necessary. Metoclopramide is the only FDA-approved prokinetic agent for gastroparesis. However, the evidence supporting its efficacy is limited, and due to its risk of serious side effects (extrapyramidal symptoms such as acute dystonic reactions, drug-induced parkinsonism, and tardive dyskinesia), its long-term use (>12 weeks) is no longer recommended by the FDA or the European Medicines Agency (EMA). Its use should be restricted to severe cases unresponsive to other therapies [54].

Other treatment options include domperidone and erythromycin, which are only effective for short-term use due to the development of tachyphylaxis [55, 56]. Gastric electrical stimulation using an implantable surgical device has received FDA approval, though its efficacy varies, and it is limited to patients with severe, refractory symptoms [57].

6. Treatment of erectile dysfunction

In addition to treating hypogonadism (if present), erectile dysfunction (ED) treatments include PDE-5 inhibitors, intracorporeal or intraurethral prostaglandins, vacuum devices, or penile prostheses.

First-line treatment consists of risk factor modification and optimization of glycemic control, sometimes requiring intensive antidiabetic therapy. In organic erectile dysfunction, sexual counseling is essential, considering the psychological impact. Treatment options include oral and local agents [28].

- Sildenafil – An oral erectogenic agent that acts peripherally on cavernous smooth muscle. It is effective even in patients with poor glycemic control or autonomic neuropathy.
    - o Adverse effects: Headache, facial flushing, dyspepsia.
    - o Contraindications: Concomitant nitrate therapy, as it increases the risk of hypotension.

- Phentolamine (Vasomax) – A non-selective alpha-receptor blocker with positive effects on erectile function, especially in older men.
  - o Adverse effects: Hypertension.
- Local therapeutic agents – Intracavernosal injections or intraurethral administration of smooth muscle relaxants.
  - o Recommended for diabetic patients with cardiovascular disease or those unresponsive to oral therapy.
  - o Intracavernosal vasodilator injections have revolutionized ED treatment.
  - o Prostaglandin E1 (PGE1) is currently the most effective agent, with rare side effects such as penile fibrosis and priapism.
- Vacuum devices – Induce erection by trapping blood in the cavernous bodies, maintained using an external constriction ring at the base of the penis.

In refractory cases, surgical penile reconstruction may be performed. Revascularization surgery involves bypassing the inferior epigastric artery to the dorsal penile artery, increasing arterial blood flow to the cavernous bodies [58].

7. Treatment of urinary dysfunction

The management of diabetic cystopathy focuses on:

- Improving continence
- Facilitating bladder emptying in retention cases
- Treating urinary tract infections

For atonic bladder with increased capacity, scheduled voiding every 3–4 hours is necessary, aiming to void a constant volume of ~400–500 mL.

In cases of high residual bladder volume, 4–5 catheterizations per day may be needed, and in some cases, permanent catheterization is required. Unfortunately, these interventions do not alter the underlying pathology but can improve the quality of life.

8. Treatment of ocular impairment

In early stages, neuropathy is reversible through improved glycemic control [59]. The DCCT (Diabetes Control and Complications Trial) strongly supports the advantage of intensive therapy in preventing clinical neuropathy [60].

Thus, screening for autonomic dysfunction is essential to prevent complications. Pupillary function tests may help early diagnosis of autonomic neuropathy.

9. Gaps in management and future directions

Despite advancements, several gaps remain in current management strategies:

1. *Early intervention deficiencies:* Many patients are diagnosed only after significant nerve damage has occurred.

2. *Limited disease-modifying treatments:* Most therapies focus on symptom relief rather than halting disease progression.

3. *Cost and accessibility barriers:* Advanced diagnostics and newer treatments remain inaccessible to many patients.

4. *Integration of AI: AI integration in neuropathy detection and prognosis*

Artificial intelligence (AI) is increasingly being integrated into the detection and prognosis of diabetic neuropathy, significantly enhancing diagnostic accuracy and patient monitoring. AI-driven algorithms have demonstrated high efficacy in analyzing retinal images to identify early vascular and structural changes associated with neuropathy, improving early diagnosis and risk stratification. These deep-learning models have been successfully applied in screening programs to detect subclinical neuropathic changes before clinical symptoms manifest [61].

Another major advancement is the application of AI in evaluating screening tools such as the Michigan Neuropathy Screening Instrument (MNSI). AI models can analyze patient-reported symptoms and clinical findings to predict the severity and progression of diabetic polyneuropathy, aiding in more effective treatment planning [62].

Furthermore, digital platforms such as Diabeta incorporate AI algorithms to streamline workflow for healthcare providers, optimize treatment plans, and enhance patient engagement. These AI-driven platforms help reduce diagnostic errors and provide real-time, personalized recommendations for managing diabetic neuropathy.

The integration of AI in diabetic neuropathy management has shown promising results, but widespread clinical adoption requires further validation through large-scale studies. Continued research is essential to enhance AI's predictive capabilities and ensure equitable access to these innovative technologies.

10. Conclusions

Diabetic neuropathy is a complication of diabetes mellitus that may be asymptomatic in up to 50% of cases, yet has a high prevalence and significantly impacts patients' quality of life.

This condition is associated with various complications, including neuropathic pain, trophic changes, and neurovegetative dysfunctions, such as ulcerations, Charcot foot, and amputations. These complications remain challenging to treat, requiring personalized approaches and multidisciplinary teams for effective management.

Prevention remains the most effective strategy, emphasizing optimal metabolic control and patient education to promote early recognition of sensory decline, including diabetic foot prophylaxis.

Acknowledgements

The authors received no financial support for this chapter's research, authorship, and publication. I confirm that I used an AI tool exclusively for the translation of the manuscript from Romanian into English, as well as for formatting the bibliography according to the publisher's requirements. All scientific content, including the analysis and interpretation, was developed independently based on national guidelines and relevant literature.

Conflict of interest

The authors declare no conflict of interest.

Author details

Andra-Elena Nica[1*], Oana Andreea Parliteanu[2], Sivu Claudia[1], Carmen Dobjanschi[1], Emilia Rusu[1] and Gabriela Radulian[1]

1 Diabetes and Endocrinology, Carol Davila University of Medicine and Pharmacy, Bucharest, ROU

2 Ambulatory, Marius Nasta Institute of Pneumology, Bucharest, ROU

*Address all correspondence to: dr.andranica@yahoo.com

References

[1] Dillon BR, Callaghan BC, Feldman EL, et al. Spectrum of diabetic neuropathy: New insights in diagnosis and treatment. Annual Review of Medicine. 2024;**75**:293-306. DOI: 10.1146/annurev-med-043021-033114

[2] Tian Z, Zhang J, Fan Y, et al. Diabetic peripheral neuropathy detection of type 2 diabetes using machine learning from TCM features: A cross-sectional study. BMC Medical Informatics and Decision Making. 2025;**25**:90. DOI: 10.1186/s12911-025-02932-w

[3] Pop-Busui R, Boulton A, Feldman EL, et al. Diabetic neuropathy: A position statement by the American Diabetes Association. Diabetes Care. 2019;**40**:136-154. DOI: 10.1038/s41572-019-0092-1

[4] Liu X, Xu Y, An M, Zen Q. The risk factors for diabetic peripheral neuropathy: A meta-analysis. PLoS One. 2019;**14**(2):e0212574. DOI: 10.1371/journal.pone.0212574

[5] Khan RMM, Chua ZJY, Tan JC, et al. From prediabetes to diabetes: Diagnosis, treatments and translational research. Medicina. 2019;**55**(9):546. DOI: 10.3390/medicina55090546

[6] Singh A, Chauhan A, Goyal P, Ramesh P. Neuropathy in prediabetics: Is oxidative stress to contribute? Journal of the Association of Physicians of India. 2019;**67**(9):60-64. Available from: https://pubmed.ncbi.nlm.nih.gov/31561691/

[7] Pai YW, Lin CH, Lin SY, Lee IT, Chang MH. Reconfirmation of newly discovered risk factors of diabetic peripheral neuropathy in patients with type 2 diabetes: A case-control study. PLoS One. 2019;**14**(7):e0220175. DOI: 10.1371/journal.pone.0220175

[8] Richner M, Ferreira N, Dudele A, et al. Functional and structural changes of the blood-nerve barrier in diabetic neuropathy. Frontiers in Neuroscience. 2018;**12**:1038. DOI: 10.3389/fnins.2018.01038

[9] Ristikj-Stomnaroska D, Risteska-Nejashmikj V, Papazova M. Role of inflammation in the pathogenesis of diabetic peripheral neuropathy. Open Access Macedonian Journal of Medical Sciences. 2019;**7**(14):2267-2270. DOI: 10.3889/oamjms.2019.646

[10] Zozulinska-Ziolkiewic D, Araszkiewicz A. Peripheral diabetic neuropathy: Better prevent than cure. Polish Archives of Internal Medicine. 2019;**129**(3):151-153. DOI: 10.20452/pamw.14773

[11] Pop-Busui R. What do we know and we do not know about cardiovascular autonomic neuropathy in diabetes. Journal of Cardiovascular Translational Research. 2012;**5**(4):463-478. DOI: 10.1007/s12265-012-9367-6

[12] Pfeifer MA. Autonomic neural dysfunction in recently diagnosed diabetic subjects. Diabetes Care. 1984;**7**(5):447-453. DOI: 10.2337/diacare.7.5.447

[13] Smith AG, Lessard M, Reyna S, Doudova M, Singleton JR. The diagnostic utility of Sudoscan for distal symmetric peripheral neuropathy. The Journal of Diabetic Complications. 2014;**28**:511-516. DOI: 10.1016/j.jdiacomp.2014.02.013

[14] Singleton RJ, Smith AG, Bromberg M. Increased prevalence of impaired glucose tolerance in patients with painful sensory neuropathy. Diabetes Care. 2001;**24**(8):1448-1453. DOI: 10.2337/diacare.24.8.1448

[15] Ulbrecht JS, Cavanagh PR, Caputo GM. Foot problems in diabetes: an overview. Clinical Infectious Diseases. 2004;**39**(Suppl 2):S73-S82. DOI: 10.1086/383266

[16] Lee S, Kim H, Choi S, et al. Clinical usefulness of two-site Semmes-Weinstein monofilament test for detecting diabetic peripheral neuropathy. Journal of Korean Medical Science. 2003;**18**:103-107. DOI: 10.3346/jkms.2003.18.1.103

[17] Lamontagne A, Buchthal F. Electrophysiological studies in diabetic neuropathy. Journal of Neurology, Neurosurgery and Psychiatry. 1970;**33**(4):442-452. DOI: 10.1136/jnnp.33.4.442

[18] Ponirak G, Petropoulus IN, Alam U, et al. Hypertension contributes to neuropathy in patients with type 1 diabetes. American Journal of Hypertension. 2019;**32**(8):796-803. DOI: 10.1093/ajh/hpz058

[19] Tsapas A, Liakos A, Paschos P, et al. A simple plaster for screening for diabetic neuropathy: A diagnostic test accuracy systematic review and meta-analysis. Metabolism. 2014;**63**:584-592. DOI: 10.1016/j.metabol.2013.11.019

[20] Chatzikosma G, Pafili K, Demetriou M, et al. Evaluation of sural nerve automated nerve conduction study in the diagnosis of peripheral neuropathy in patients with type 2 diabetes mellitus. Archives of Medical Science. 2016;**12**(2):390-393. DOI: 10.5114/aoms.2016.59265

[21] Pafili K, Maltezos E, Papanas N. NC-stat for the diagnosis of diabetic polyneuropathy. Expert Review of Medical Devices. 2017;**14**(4):251-254. DOI: 10.1080/17434440.2017.1305266

[22] Willits I, Cole H, Jones R, Dimmock P, Arber M. VibraTip for testing vibration perception to detect diabetic peripheral neuropathy: A NICE medical technology guidance. Applied Health Economics and Health Policy. 2015;**13**(4):315-324. DOI: 10.1007/s40258-015-0181-6

[23] Dias LS, Nienov OH, Parisi M, Schmid H. Sensitivity and specificity of neuropathy diabetes score, neuropathy symptoms score, diabetic neuropathy score and esthesiometry compared with the gold standards Michigan neuropathy screening instrument (MNSI) and Beck depression inventory (BDI). Diabetology and Metabolic Syndrome. 2015;**7**(Suppl 1):A199. DOI: 10.1186/1758-5996-7-S1-A199

[24] Standards of care in diabetes 2024, chapter retinopathy, neuropathy and foot care. Diabetes Care. 2024;**47**(Suppl 1):235. DOI: 10.2337/dc24-S012

[25] Vinik AI, Maser RE, Mitchell BD, Freeman R. Diabetic autonomic neuropathy. Diabetes Care. 2003;**26**:1553-1579. DOI: 10.2337/diacare.26.5.1553

[26] American Academy of Neurology. Assessment: Clinical autonomic testing report. Neurology. 1996;**46**(3):873-880. Available from: https://pubmed.ncbi.nlm.nih.gov/8618715/

[27] Low PA, Denq JC, Opfer-Gehrking TL, et al. Effect of age and gender on sudomotor and cardiovagal function and blood pressure response to tilt in normal subjects. Muscle & Nerve. 1997;**20**(12):1561-1568. DOI: 10.1002/(sici)1097-4598(199712)20:12<1561::aid-mus11>3.0.co;2-3

[28] Boulton AJ, Vinik AI, Arezzo JC, et al. Diabetic neuropathies: A statement by the American Diabetes Association. Diabetes Care. 2019;**28**(4):956-962. DOI: 10.2337/diacare.28.4.956

[29] American Diabetes Association. Microvascular complications and foot care: Standards of medical care in diabetes – 2019. Diabetes Care. 2019;**42**(Suppl. 1):S124-S138. DOI: 10.2337/dc19-S011

[30] Callaghan BC, Xia R, Banerjee M, et al. Metabolic syndrome components are associated with symptomatic polyneuropathy independent of glycemic status. Diabetes Care. 2016;**39**:801-807. DOI: 10.2337/dc16-0081

[31] Andersen ST, Witte DR, Dalsgaard EM, et al. Risk factors for incident diabetic polyneuropathy in a cohort with screen-detected type 2 diabetes followed for 13 years: ADDITION-Denmark. Diabetes Care. 2018;**41**:1068-1075. DOI: 10.2337/dc17-2062

[32] Lu Y, Xing P, Cai X, et al. Prevalence and risk factors for diabetic peripheral neuropathy in type 2 diabetic patients from 14 countries: Estimates of the INTERPRET-DD study. Frontiers in Public Health. 2020;**8**:534372. DOI: 10.3389/fpubh.2020.534372

[33] Tang Y, Shan H, Bueno Junior CR, et al. Intensive risk factor management and cardiovascular autonomic neuropathy in type 2 diabetes: The ACCORD trial. Diabetes Care. 2021;**44**:146-173. DOI: 10.2337/dc20-1842

[34] Shahid W, Kumar R, Shaikh A, et al. Comparison of the efficacy of duloxetine and pregabalin in pain relief associated with diabetic neuropathy. Cureus. 2019;**11**(7):e5293. DOI: 10.7759/cureus.5293

[35] Ziegler D, Hidvegi T, Guirieva I, et al. Efficacy and safety of lacosamide in painful diabetic neuropathy. Diabetes Care. 2010;**33**(4):839-841. DOI: 10.2337/dc09-1578

[36] Vinik A, Rosenstock J, Sharma U, et al. Efficacy and safety of mirogabalin (DS-5565) for the treatment of diabetic peripheral neuropathic pain: A randomized, double-blind, placebo-controlled study. Diabetes Care. 2014;**37**(12):3253-3261. DOI: 10.2337/dc14-1044

[37] Papanas N, Ziegler D. Emerging drugs for diabetic peripheral neuropathy and neuropathic pain. Expert Opinion on Emerging Drugs. 2016;**21**(4):393-407. DOI: 10.1080/14728214.2016.1257605

[38] Bramson C, Herrmann DN, Carey W, et al. Exploring the role of tanezumab as a novel treatment for the relief of neuropathic pain. Pain Medicine. 2015;**16**(6):1163-1176. DOI: 10.1111/pme.12677

[39] Price R, Smith D, Franklin G, et al. Oral and topical treatment of painful diabetic polyneuropathy: Practice guideline update summary. Neurology. 2022;**98**(1):31-34. DOI: 10.1212/WNL.0000000000013038

[40] Fonseca VA, Lavery LA, Thethi EK, et al. Metanx in type 2 diabetes with peripheral neuropathy: A randomized trial. American Journal of Medicine. 2013;**126**(2):141-149. DOI: 10.1016/j.amjmed.2012.06.022

[41] Brines M, Dunne AN, van Velzen M, Proto PL. ARA 290, a nonerythropoietic peptide engineered from erythropoietin, improves metabolic control and neuropathic symptoms in patients with type 2 diabetes. Molecular Medicine. 2015;**20**:658-666. DOI: 10.2119/molmed.2014.00215

[42] Writing Team for the Diabetes Control and Complications Trial/Epidemiology of Diabetes Interventions and Complications Research Group. Sustained effect of intensive treatment of

type 1 diabetes mellitus on development and progression of diabetic nephropathy: The EDIC study. Journal of the American Medical Association. 2003;**290**(16):2159-2167. DOI: 10.1001/jama.290.16.2159

[43] Spallone V, Ziegler D, Freeman R, et al. Cardiovascular autonomic neuropathy in diabetes: Clinical impact, assessment, diagnosis, and management. Toronto consensus panel on diabetic neuropathy. Diabetes/Metabolism Research and Reviews. 2011;**27**(7):639-653. DOI: 10.1002/dmrr.1239

[44] Martin CL, Albers JW, Pop-Busui R, DCCT/EDIC Research Group. Neuropathy and related findings in the DCCT/EDIC study. Diabetes Care. 2014;**37**:31-38. DOI: 10.2337/dc13-2114

[45] Gaede P, Oellgaard J, Carstensen B, et al. Years of life gained by multifactorial intervention in patients with type 2 diabetes mellitus and microalbuminuria: 21 years follow-up on the Steno-2 randomized trial. Diabetologia. 2016;**59**:2298-2307. DOI: 10.1007/s00125-016-4065-6

[46] Gibbons CH, Schmidt P, Biaggioni I, et al. The recommendations of a consensus panel for the screening, diagnosis, and treatment of neurogenic orthostatic hypotension and associated supine hypertension. Journal of Neurology. 2017;**264**:1567-1582. DOI: 10.1007/s00415-016-8375-x

[47] Standards of care in diabetes 2024, chapter retinopathy, neuropathy and foot care. Diabetes Care. 2024;**47**(Suppl 1):237. DOI: 10.2337/dc24-S012

[48] Briasoulis A, Silver A, Yano Y, Bakris GL. Orthostatic hypotension associated with baroreceptor dysfunction: Treatment approaches. Journal of Clinical Hypertension. 2014;**16**:141-148. DOI: 10.1111/jch.12258

[49] Figueroa JJ, Basford JR, Low PA. Preventing and treating orthostatic hypotension: as easy as a, B, C. Cleveland Clinic Journal of Medicine. 2010;**77**:298-306. DOI: 10.3949/ccjm.77a.09118

[50] Jordan J, Fanciulli A, Tank J, et al. Management of supine hypertension in patients with neurogenic orthostatic hypotension: Scientific statement of the American autonomic society, European Federation of Autonomic Societies, and the European Society of Hypertension. Journal of Hypertension. 2019;**37**:1541-1546. DOI: 10.1097/HJH.0000000000002078

[51] Brignole M, Moya A, de Lange FJ, et al. 2018 ESC guidelines for the diagnosis and management of syncope. European Heart Journal. 2019;**39**(21):1883-1948. DOI: 10.1093/eurheartj/ehy037

[52] Camilleri M, Parkman HP, Shafi MA, Abell TL, Gerson L, American College of Gastroenterology. Clinical guideline: Management of gastroparesis. American Journal of Gastroenterology. 2013;**108**:18-37. DOI: 10.1038/ajg.2012.373

[53] Parrish CR, Pastors JG. Nutritional management of gastroparesis in people with diabetes. Diabetes Spectrum. 2007;**20**:231-234. DOI: 10.2337/diaspect.20.4.231

[54] Pop-Busui R, Stevens M. Autonomic neuropathy in diabetes. In: Umpierrez GE, editor. Therapy for Diabetes Mellitus and Related Disorders. 6th ed. Alexandria, VA: American Diabetes Association; 2014. pp. 834-864. ISBN Print: 978-1-58040-509-6

[55] Maganti K, Onyemere K, Jones MP. Oral erythromycin and symptomatic relief of gastroparesis: A systematic review. American Journal of Gastroenterology. 2003;**98**:259-263. DOI: 10.1111/j.1572-0241.2003.07167.x

[56] McCallum RW, Snape W, Brody F, et al. Gastric electrical stimulation with enterra therapy improves symptoms from diabetic gastroparesis in a prospective study. Clinical Gastroenterology and Hepatology. 2010;**8**:947-954. DOI: 10.1016/j.cgh.2010.05.020

[57] Vinik AI. Advances in diabetes for the millennium: New treatments for diabetic neuropathies. MedGenMed. 2014;**6**(2):13-17. Available from: https://pmc.ncbi.nlm.nih.gov/articles/PMC1474828/

[58] Donaghue KC. Autonomic neuropathy: Diagnosis and impact on health in adolescents with diabetes. Hormone Research. 2008;**50**:33-37. DOI: 10.1159/000053100

[59] Lanting P, Strijers RL, Bos JE, Faes TJ, Heimans JJ. The cause of increased light reflex latencies in diabetic patients: The relationship between pupillary light reflex and visual evoked potential latencies. Electroencephalography and Clinical Neurophysiology. 1999;**78**:111-115. DOI: 10.1016/0013-4694(91)90110-p

[60] Radu R, Radulian G. Neuropatiile diabetice. In: Radulian G, editor. Diabetul Zaharat în Practica Medicală. Bucharest: Carol Davila University Press; 2019. pp. 124-147. ISBN: 978-606-011-060-6

[61] Yang Q, Bee YM, Lim CC, Sabanayagam C, Yim-Lui Cheung C, Wong TY, et al. Use of artificial intelligence with retinal imaging in screening for diabetes-associated complications: Systematic review. EClinicalMedicine. 2025;**81**:103089. DOI: 10.1016/j.eclinm.2025.103089

[62] Haque F, Reaz MB, Chowdhury ME, Malik R, Alhatou M, Kobashi S, et al. A machine learning-based severity prediction tool for diabetic sensorimotor polyneuropathy using Michigan neuropathy screening instrumentations. arXiv preprint arXiv:2203.15151. 2022. DOI: 10.48550/arXiv.2203.15151

Section 4

Chemotherapy-Induced Neuropathies

Chapter 4

Integrated Approaches to Managing Cancer Treatment-Induced Peripheral Neuropathies: Risk Factors, Interventions, and Clinical Pathways

Sébastien S. Dufresne, Pauline Jardel, Mélanie Brassard, Patricia Bilodeau and Edith De Grand'Maison

Abstract

This chapter presents an in-depth exploration of peripheral neuropathy as a frequent and often persistent complication associated with cancer treatments, including chemotherapy, immunotherapy, and radiotherapy. Rather than limiting the discussion to descriptive aspects, the text engages with the underlying mechanisms that contribute to neurotoxicity, establishing a dynamic link between molecular alterations and clinical expression. In addressing management strategies, the chapter integrates both pharmacological and non-pharmacological interventions, each critically examined within the context of current scientific evidence and clinical applicability. A particular focus is placed on the identification of early risk indicators, such as metabolic dysregulation, prior neurological conditions, and modifiable lifestyle behaviors, that collectively influence patient susceptibility and therapeutic response. The analysis further incorporates the specificities of radiation-induced neuropathies, acknowledging their distinct pathophysiological trajectory while embedding them within an overarching management continuum. To facilitate the translation of theoretical knowledge into clinical decision-making, a structured algorithm is proposed, intended to support the development of personalized, integrative treatment pathways that address not only symptom relief but also long-term neurofunctional preservation and overall patient well-being.

Keywords: cancer treatment-induced peripheral neuropathy, pharmacological interventions, non-pharmacological interventions, risk factor modification, clinical pathway

1. Introduction

Peripheral neuropathy (PN) is a prevalent and frequently disabling consequence of cancer treatment, characterized by a heterogeneous array of sensory, motor, and autonomic symptoms that can persist long after therapy completion [1, 2]. While it is most commonly associated with cytotoxic chemotherapy, PN is increasingly recognized across a broader therapeutic landscape, including radiotherapy and immunotherapy [3]. Its manifestations, ranging from paresthesia and dysesthesia to balance impairment and fine motor dysfunction, can significantly impact patients' autonomy, safety, and quality of life [4]. More than a side effect, PN has become a clinically significant factor influencing treatment intensity, functional outcomes, and survivorship planning.

Epidemiological data underscore the scope of the problem. Neuropathy affects a substantial proportion of patients undergoing neurotoxic regimens, with prevalence estimates varying widely depending on treatment class, cumulative dose, and individual susceptibility [1, 5–7]. In certain populations, including older adults and individuals with pre-existing vulnerabilities, symptoms may persist for months or years after treatment, reflecting the potential for chronic nerve injury [8, 9]. Despite this burden, PN remains in routine clinical practice, and the discrepancy between patient-reported symptoms and clinician documentation is well documented [10]. The spectrum of treatments associated with PN is expanding. Well-established chemotherapeutic agents, such as platinum salts, taxanes, and vinca alkaloids, are known for their dose-limiting neurotoxicity [11]. Newer classes, including proteasome inhibitors and immunomodulatory agents, also contribute to peripheral nerve injury, albeit through different mechanisms [11–13]. Moreover, the resurgence of immune checkpoint inhibitors (ICIs) has brought attention to a set of rare but potentially severe immune-mediated neuropathies [14, 15]. Radiation-induced neuropathies, historically overlooked, constitute another unique category of nerve injury, characterized by their insidious onset and progressive nature [16]. These treatment-specific pathways and mechanisms will be analyzed in detail later in the chapter.

Functionally, PN undermines patients' ability to engage in daily activities and is associated with increased fall risk, emotional distress, and long-term functional decline [17]. Clinically, it may necessitate treatment delays, dose reductions, or discontinuation, altering therapeutic trajectories and, in some cases, compromising oncologic outcomes [18, 19]. Still, standardized approaches for risk stratification, early detection, and longitudinal management remain limited. Although several individual risk factors have been identified, ranging from age and metabolic status to prior neurological disease, no predictive algorithm has yet gained widespread clinical adoption [20]. Therapeutic options remain suboptimal. While some pharmacologic agents have demonstrated symptomatic benefit, none have shown convincing evidence of disease-modifying effects. Non-pharmacological interventions are emerging as promising adjuncts, but their integration into standard care remains uneven across practice settings [21].

This chapter offers an integrated and interdisciplinary perspective on treatment-induced peripheral neuropathies, structured around key clinical and mechanistic domains. It begins by exploring the biological underpinnings of neurotoxicity across cancer therapies, before addressing the factors that modulate individual vulnerability. The clinical presentation of PN is then examined in relation to neuroanatomical targets and treatment-specific features, followed by a critical analysis of available therapeutic strategies. Special focus is given to underrecognized forms such as radiation-induced neuropathies.

Throughout the chapter, the term *treatment-induced peripheral neuropathy* (TIPN) is used as an umbrella term encompassing neuropathic complications resulting from cancer therapies, including chemotherapy, immunotherapy, and radiotherapy.

DOI: http://dx.doi.org/10.5772/intechopen.1011121

When referring specifically to chemotherapy-related mechanisms, we use the term *chemotherapy-induced peripheral neuropathy* (CIPN), while *radiation-induced peripheral neuropathy* (RIPN) is used in contexts involving regional radiotherapy. The broader abbreviation peripheral neuropathy (*PN*) is reserved for general references to clinical symptoms or outcomes that are not linked to a specific treatment modality. This terminological framework is applied consistently throughout the chapter to promote clarity and conceptual precision across disciplines. Drawing on this foundation, the chapter proposes a stratified clinical framework to support personalized decision-making. Finally, it looks ahead to innovations in monitoring, neuroregeneration, and survivorship-oriented care.

2. Distinct mechanisms and shared outcomes: Neuropathy across treatment modalities

PN induced by cancer therapies represents a clinically heterogeneous entity underpinned by diverse yet partially overlapping pathophysiological processes. As illustrated in **Figure 1**, peripheral nerve damage can involve axonal transport disruption, mitochondrial dysfunction, ion channel dysregulation, inflammatory responses, glial activation, microtubule destabilization, ischemia, and progressive fibrosis. While these mechanisms vary according to therapeutic class, their cumulative clinical expression converges around a shared symptomatology, typically involving sensory-dominant, distal-predominant neuropathies.

2.1 Chemotherapy-induced peripheral neuropathy (CIPN)

CIPN is driven by agent-specific neurotoxic mechanisms, often targeting dorsal root ganglia (DRG) sensory neurons [22]. The clinical phenotype is generally length-dependent and sensory-dominant, though motor and autonomic components may also emerge depending on the regimen and cumulative dose [23]. The biological injury profile reflects the molecular characteristics of the cytotoxic agent, making

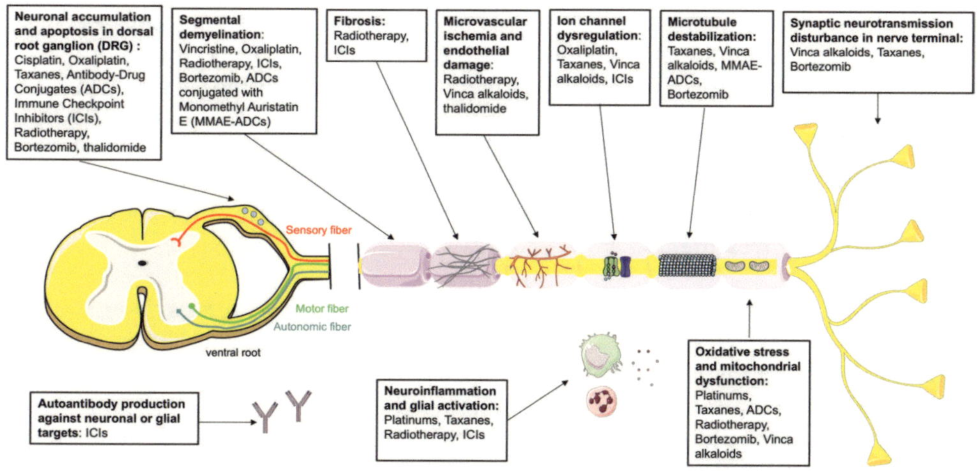

Figure 1.
Mechanisms of cancer treatment-induced peripheral neuropathy across neural compartments.

mechanistic discrimination essential for anticipating symptom onset and tailoring mitigation strategies. Microtubule-stabilizing agents, particularly taxanes such as paclitaxel and docetaxel, promote neurotoxicity by disrupting the physiological dynamics of microtubule assembly [12, 23, 24]. By locking microtubules into a rigid, non-dynamic state, these agents interfere with mitochondrial trafficking, vesicle transport, and axonal signaling, culminating in intra-axonal congestion and distal axon degeneration [13]. Paclitaxel further activates Toll-like receptor 4 (TLR4) in DRG macrophages, triggering the release of inflammatory cytokines (e.g., TNF-α, IL-1β) that enhance nociceptor sensitivity and perpetuate pain signaling [11]. Platinum salts, such as cisplatin and oxaliplatin, cause nerve damage mainly by forming harmful bonds with DNA (called DNA adducts) and by increasing oxidative stress in mitochondria [22, 25]. These changes trigger cell death (apoptosis) in neurons of the DRG through mechanisms involving the p53 protein, and they also reduce the ability of mitochondria to produce energy by allowing the accumulation of toxic molecules known as reactive oxygen species [11, 26]. Oxaliplatin, in particular, has been linked to abnormal sensitivity to cold (cold-induced dysesthesias), which is thought to result from its effects on specific ion channels, including sodium (NaV1.6), TRPA1, TRPM8, and potassium channels. This points to a direct disruption on the way electrical signals are transmitted in sensory nerves [4, 27]. Proteasome inhibitors, especially bortezomib, damage nerves through a different mechanism. They disrupt the cell's ability to manage proteins properly (proteostatic stress) and interfere with calcium channels that regulate nerve activity. This leads to a chain reaction involving stress in the endoplasmic reticulum, swelling of mitochondria, a drop in available cellular energy (ATP depletion), and ultimately a breakdown in the structure of nerve fibers [1, 13]. Clinically, neuropathy caused by bortezomib shows signs of both axonal damage and demyelination, suggesting that multiple parts of the nerve cell are affected, not just the axon itself [1, 13, 28]. Vinca alkaloids such as vincristine interfere with tubulin polymerization, causing mitotic arrest and cytoskeletal breakdown. Their toxicity primarily affects large myelinated fibers and leads to combined sensory, motor, and autonomic symptoms [1, 11, 28]. These agents also disrupt axonal continuity and show heightened neurotoxicity in children and in patients with predisposing risk factors [26].

In addition to direct neuronal damage, non-neuronal cells also play a key role in PN. Chemotherapy activates satellite glial cells, microglia, and macrophages, which release inflammatory molecules such as CCL2 and IL-6. These mediators increase nerve sensitivity in both the peripheral and central nervous systems [29]. Regardless of the drug class, many agents lead to mitochondrial dysfunction. This includes the loss of membrane potential, disrupted calcium balance, and the release of cytochrome c, all of which contribute to energy failure and axonal damage [13]. These mitochondrial alterations may help explain why neuropathy often persists well beyond the end of treatment.

2.2 Immune-associated neuropathies and antibody-drug conjugates

Immune checkpoint inhibitors (ICIs), such as nivolumab, pembrolizumab, atezolizumab, and ipilimumab, have revolutionized oncology but can also elicit immune-mediated neuropathies. These are rare but often severe and include conditions such as Guillain-Barré syndrome (GBS), chronic inflammatory demyelinating polyradiculoneuropathy (CIDP), and sensory neuronopathies [14]. Pharmacovigilance studies have confirmed these associations. In the FAERS database, Mikami et al. identified 204 cases of ICI-induced PN, with the highest reporting odds for anti-PD-1 agents [14]. Combination regimens further increased the risk of neurologic immune-related adverse events. Using data from the WHO pharmacovigilance database (VigiBase), Johnson et al. identified over 560 cases of peripheral neuropathy associated with immune checkpoint inhibitors (ICIs), including Guillain-Barré syndrome (GBS, 22% of cases), chronic polyneuropathies, and mononeuropathies [30]. The median onset varied by syndrome, with GBS typically occurring within 66 days of treatment initiation. Fatality rates ranged from 10% to 20%, with the highest mortality observed in patients with myasthenia gravis. Mechanistically, ICIs can cause nerve damage by interfering with the body's normal mechanisms that prevent the immune system from attacking its own tissues. This loss of immune control can lead to inflammation and damage in the peripheral nervous system, including the protective myelin around nerves and structures such as the dorsal root ganglia [30]. A related issue is seen with antibody-drug conjugates (ADCs), especially those that include a compound called monomethyl auristatin E (MMAE), like enfortumab vedotin [31]. Even though these treatments are designed to target cancer cells specifically, MMAE affects the internal structure of nerve cells in a way similar to taxanes, leading to nerve damage that mostly affects sensory function. Preclinical and FAERS data show a high neuropathy signal (ROR = 6.45), involving distal axonopathy, demyelination, and conduction block [31]. These neuropathies sit at the intersection of immune toxicity and classical cytoskeletal disruption, highlighting the need for precise etiological attribution and tailored therapeutic responses.

2.3 Radiation-induced peripheral neuropathy (RIPN)

RIPN is a delayed, often underrecognized complication of regional radiotherapy. All peripheral nerves may be affected, depending on the anatomical site of radiation delivery. For example, pelvic irradiation may involve the lumbosacral plexus, while supraclavicular radiation can damage the brachial plexus. Critically, all tissues within the irradiated field are potentially susceptible to injury, with risk increasing as a function of total dose, fraction size, and irradiated volume.

Radiotherapy planning involves a constant balancing act between oncologic efficacy and normal tissue preservation. The guiding principle for organs at risk (OARs) is ALARA, "as low as reasonably achievable," yet this must often yield to the imperative of tumor control. To mediate this tension, dose-volume constraints are employed to minimize the likelihood of severe toxicity. For instance, in stereotactic ablative radiotherapy (SABR), the maximum-tolerated dose to the brachial plexus is approximately 15 Gy in a single fraction, 32 Gy in five fractions, or 39 Gy in eight fractions, according to the British consensus on SABR planning [32]. In conventional fractionation (1.8–2 Gy per fraction), the upper limit for peripheral nerves is generally considered to be around 55–60 Gy, beyond which the probability of irreversible neurologic damage markedly increases.

SABR techniques rely on submillimetric precision, high conformality, and steep dose gradients to spare adjacent OARs. Peripheral nerves behave as functionally serial structures, where injury to a single segment can cause global dysfunction. This stands in contrast to parallel organs (e.g., liver), where function depends on the volume of spared subunits. Accurate anatomical delineation of nervous structures is therefore imperative, especially in reirradiation scenarios where cumulative dose must be carefully assessed. Atlas-based contouring guidelines have been developed to aid in this process.

Pathophysiologically, RIPN reflects a triad of direct neural damage, ischemia, and progressive fibrosis. Early effects include DNA strand breaks, myelin vacuolization, and capillary rarefaction, while chronic injury is marked by fibroblast activation, collagen deposition, and perineural scarring. These changes result in mechanical compression and irreversible axonal loss [33, 34]. Histological findings typically reveal axonal dropout, segmental demyelination, and fibrotic encapsulation. MRI may demonstrate T2-weighted hyperintensities or contrast enhancement, although clinical-radiologic correlation remains essential.

Due to its gradual and insidious course, RIPN is frequently misdiagnosed as tumor recurrence or degenerative disease, delaying appropriate recognition [33]. Unlike chemotherapy- or immune-related neuropathies, RIPN is non-inflammatory and fibrotic in nature, posing distinct challenges for prevention and therapeutic intervention.

3. From risk to reality: Identifying patients at the edge

The onset of TIPN is rarely the sole consequence of pharmacological exposure. Instead, it arises from a dynamic interaction between the neurotoxic potential of antineoplastic agents and a patient's intrinsic vulnerability. This vulnerability is shaped by a network of predisposing, precipitating, and perpetuating factors, encompassing prior neurological conditions, metabolic status, genetic variability, and modifiable lifestyle parameters [35]. Understanding these factors is essential for risk stratification, anticipatory monitoring, and early intervention.

Among the most consistent predisposing elements are pre-existing neuropathic conditions, including diabetic polyneuropathy, HIV-associated neuropathy, hereditary sensory-motor neuropathies, and chronic entrapment syndromes [8, 20, 36, 37]. These disorders create a pro-neuropathic terrain *via* sustained low-grade inflammation, maladaptive ion channel expression, and microvascular compromise, effectively lowering the threshold for neurotoxic injury upon chemotherapy or immunotherapy exposure [9, 38]. Metabolic dysregulation further exacerbates susceptibility. Obesity, dyslipidemia, insulin resistance, and elevated fasting glucose have each been linked to more severe or earlier-onset TIPN, particularly in patients treated with platinum agents or taxanes [9, 20]. In parallel, micronutrient deficiencies, notably in vitamin B12 and vitamin D, impair axonal repair mechanisms, heighten oxidative stress, and compromise neuroprotection [39–42]. While chronological age is frequently cited as a risk factor, evidence suggests that functional markers, such as frailty, anemia, or sarcopenia, may offer greater predictive value [9]. Mizrahi et al. [9], in a prospective study of 333 patients receiving taxanes or platinum salts, demonstrated that older age, lower baseline hemoglobin, and higher body mass index (BMI) independently predicted neuropathy severity. Specifically, lower hemoglobin levels ($\beta = -0.47$; $p < .001$), higher BMI ($\beta = 0.08$; $p = .007$), and older age ($\beta = 0.08$; $p < .001$) were all associated with increased total neuropathy scores. These variables also correlated with worse performance on functional assessments such as two-point discrimination and fine motor dexterity tests, indicating that clinical burden extends beyond subjective symptoms.

The role of pharmacogenetics is increasingly acknowledged, though not yet implemented in clinical practice. Polymorphisms in genes involved in drug metabolism (e.g., CYP2C8), ion channel structure (e.g., SCN9A), and microtubule dynamics (e.g., CEP72) have been linked to heightened TIPN risk in patients receiving agents such as vincristine, paclitaxel, or oxaliplatin [25, 26, 29, 40, 43]. These findings highlight interindividual differences in neuronal resilience and pave the way for future personalized medicine approaches.

Concomitant medications can also modulate neuropathy risk. Observational data suggest that beta-blockers may aggravate TIPN, potentially *via* compromised peripheral perfusion [44], whereas calcium channel blockers and renin-angiotensin system inhibitors may have neutral or even protective effects. Some statins and antiretroviral therapies have also been implicated, underscoring the importance of comprehensive medication review in patients undergoing neurotoxic regimens [20]. Lifestyle-related variables, while often underemphasized, are modifiable determinants of neuropathic vulnerability. Tobacco and alcohol use contribute to mitochondrial dysfunction and impaired axonal regeneration, while sedentary behavior fosters systemic inflammation and altered neurovascular coupling [45]. Conversely, observational studies show that patients engaging in more than 5 hours per week of moderate-to-vigorous physical activity exhibit a significantly lower risk of persistent TIPN symptoms [25, 46].

Although intrinsic factors are central, cumulative treatment exposure remains a key determinant. For agents such as oxaliplatin and paclitaxel, neuropathy severity scales with total dose. However, adaptive strategies such as *stop-and-go* regimens have shown potential in reducing progression to high-grade TIPN without compromising treatment efficacy [47]. In study by Relias et al., intermittent treatment schedules allowed partial symptom regression and minimized chronicity, highlighting the feasibility of dynamic treatment modulation [47].

Ultimately, TIPN susceptibility is multifactorial and synergistic. Single-risk factors rarely explain interindividual differences; rather, it is the accumulation and interaction of biological, behavioral, and treatment-related variables that shape the clinical outcomes. This reinforces the need to evolve from agent-centric approaches to integrate risk models that inform preventive strategies, monitoring intensity, and escalation thresholds in oncologic care.

4. The clinical spectrum: When nerves speak

4.1 Patterns of presentation: Acute, chronic, and coasting syndromes

The clinical presentation of TIPN is shaped not only by the pharmacological class of the antineoplastic agent but also by the anatomical and physiological characteristics of the affected nerve fibers. **Table 1** provides a structured typology of peripheral nerve fibers grouped by sensory, motor, and autonomic functions and highlights their respective levels of myelination, conduction velocity, and clinical implications when damaged. This classification supports diagnostic reasoning by linking fiber subtype involvement to specific patterns of symptoms, such as burning pain, proprioceptive deficits, or autonomic instability.

Platinum compounds exemplify the heterogeneity of TIPN manifestations. Oxaliplatin frequently induces a distinct, short-latency syndrome marked by cold-induced paresthesia, fasciculations, and perioral dysesthesia within hours of infusion. This acute response, reported in many patients, reflects transient hyperexcitability of dorsal root ganglion neurons triggered by oxalate metabolites and sodium channel dysfunction [25]. Although reversible between cycles, its intensity may predict the onset of chronic sensory neuropathy, which typically

Fiber types		Main roles	Typical clinical manifestation if altered	Known vulnerability	Justification
Sensory	Aα – Ia 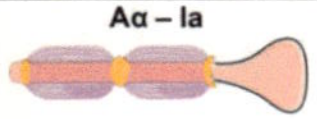	Detection of muscle length change; initiation of stretch reflex	Hyporeflexia, sensory ataxia, imbalance	High	Large-diameter, heavily myelinated Ia afferents are located in the DRG and are selectively vulnerable to cisplatin and oxaliplatin due to platinum accumulation and DNA adduct formation, leading to apoptotic loss of proprioceptive neurons and disruption of stretch reflex pathways.
	Aα – Ib 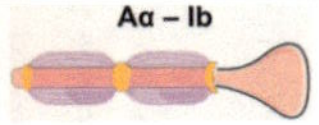	Monitoring of muscle tension; inhibition of excessive contraction	Loss of tendon reflexes, poor load adaptation	Moderate to high	Ib afferents share a similar vulnerability profile to Ia fibers through platinum-induced DRG toxicity. Their involvement in Golgi tendon feedback loops is disrupted by neuronal apoptosis and inflammatory signaling.
	Aβ 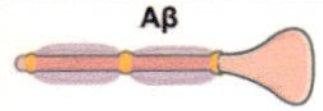	Discriminative touch, vibration, and conscious proprioception	Numbness, loss of fine touch, imbalance	High	Aβ fibers are myelinated and large-caliber, making them highly susceptible to mitochondrial dysfunction, disruption of ion channel conductance, and demyelination. These effects are induced by taxanes, bortezomib, and platinum agents, resulting in tactile and proprioceptive deficits.
	Aδ 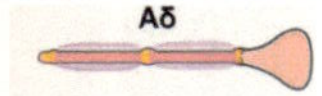	Rapid detection of noxious mechanical and thermal stimuli	Reduced sharp pain, cold dysesthesia, cold hypersensitivity	Moderate	Aδ fibers are selectively targeted by oxaliplatin through modulation of voltage-gated sodium channels (NaV1.6) and TRP channels (TRPA1, TRPM8), causing cold dysesthesia and reduced mechanical nociception. Taxanes contribute through microglial activation and cytokine-mediated sensitization.
	C 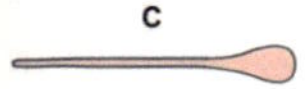	Slow pain signaling, thermal sensitivity, itch perception	Burning pain, allodynia, chronic discomfort	High	C fibers, due to their unmyelinated and metabolically active profile, are highly susceptible to mitochondrial stress, ROS generation, and glial-mediated neuroinflammation. Chronic exposure to platinum agents, radiation, and ICI-related cytokine storms amplifies sensory neuron degeneration and dysfunctional pain signaling.

DOI: http://dx.doi.org/10.5772/intechopen.1011121

Fiber types		Main roles	Typical clinical manifestation if altered	Known vulnerability	Justification
Motor	Aα 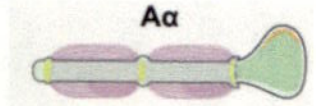	Activation of skeletal muscle for voluntary movement	Distal weakness, cramps, atrophy	Low to moderate	Motor Aα fibers are affected by agents disrupting cytoskeletal integrity such as vincristine and MMAE-ADCs. These treatments impair axonal transport *via* microtubule destabilization, leading to distal axonopathy and muscle weakness. Radiation may add ischemic or fibrotic injury to motor roots.
	Aγ 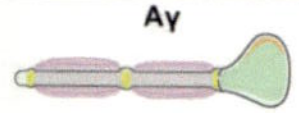	Modulation of muscle spindle sensitivity to stretch	Stiffness, impaired tone adjustment	Unknown	Though direct evidence is scarce, Aγ fibers are likely affected in mixed sensory-motor neuropathies. Cytoskeletal and inflammatory alterations may impair intrafusal fiber regulation, contributing to fine motor instability.
Autonomic	B fibers 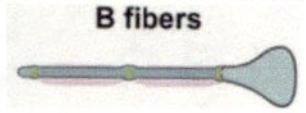	Sympathetic output to autonomic ganglia (preganglionic)	Orthostatic hypotension, pupillary changes	Moderate	B fibers are lightly myelinated preganglionic autonomic neurons. They are impaired by immune-related inflammation and radiation-induced ganglionopathy, leading to dysautonomia *via* sympathetic tone loss.
	C autonomic 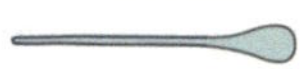	Autonomic regulation of visceral and glandular targets	Dry mouth, thermal dysregulation, GI dysmotility	High	C autonomic fibers are small and unmyelinated, mediating visceral autonomic responses. They are damaged by cytokine-mediated neurotoxicity (ICI), oxidative stress, and chronic metabolic dysregulation, resulting in glandular and gastrointestinal autonomic failure.

Table 1.
Peripheral nerve fiber types and their vulnerabilities to cancer treatment-induced neuropathy.

emerges after cumulative doses surpassing 780–850 mg/m^2 and manifests as proprioceptive loss, distal hypoesthesia, and delayed coasting phenomena [9, 48]. Cisplatin, while less associated with acute syndromes, produces a similar chronic axonal neuropathy targeting large-diameter sensory fibers, with glove-and-stocking distribution, vibration loss, and gait disturbance, features correlated with DNA repair capacity and adduct burden [12, 23, 24].

Taxanes, particularly paclitaxel, may cause an early-onset musculoskeletal "acute pain syndrome" within 72 hours, involving deep aching in the back and limbs, which resolves within a week [6, 19]. Chronic taxane neuropathy develops insidiously and exhibits a length-dependent, symmetric profile affecting both small and large fibers, with symptoms of numbness, tingling, and proprioceptive impairment that can persist for months or years [8, 37, 49]. Vinca alkaloids such as vincristine induce a mixed neuropathy often evident after the first cycle. Motor symptoms, including distal weakness and foot drop, may precede sensory changes, while autonomic signs such as orthostatic hypotension and urinary retention are not uncommon. Neurotoxicity may persist well beyond treatment, particularly in pediatric populations, in whom long-term motor deficits are observed [1, 11, 13, 43]. Proteasome inhibitors such as bortezomib typically result in small-fiber neuropathies, manifesting as burning pain, allodynia, and stocking-glove sensory loss. While some patients recover within 3 months post-treatment, 30–40% may experience lasting symptoms. Mechanistically, these neuropathies reflect mitochondrial dysfunction and apoptosis in dorsal root ganglia.

Thalidomide and related immunomodulatory drugs cause predominantly irreversible, length-dependent axonopathies with sensory and occasional cranial or autonomic involvement [1, 11, 12, 28]. In contrast, antibody-drug conjugates (e.g., brentuximab vedotin), which couple monoclonal antibodies with cytotoxic agents such as monomethyl auristatin E, produce irreversible sensory neuropathies driven by microtubule disruption, particularly in patients with prior chemotherapy exposure or predisposing factors [31]. Immune checkpoint inhibitors (ICIs), including PD-1, PD-L1, and CTLA-4 inhibitors, induce autoimmune neuropathies that are typically acute or subacute and not dose-dependent. These syndromes, such as Guillain-Barré syndrome, chronic inflammatory demyelinating polyradiculoneuropathy, or sensory neuronopathy, are often asymmetric and multifocal, and may not resolve without the immunomodulatory treatment.

4.2 Clinical detection and multimodal assessment strategies

Despite growing awareness of neurotoxicity in oncology, TIPNs are frequently underdiagnosed or mischaracterized. The diagnostic approach must therefore integrate clinical, patient-reported, and objective findings. In real-world settings, symptom detection often relies on patient self-report and basic neurological testing [50, 51]. However, vague descriptors such as "tingling" or "numbness" lack diagnostic precision and may delay intervention [48]. Standard grading tools like CTCAE offer limited granularity and are poorly sensitive to subclinical deficits [8].

Validated instruments such as the total neuropathy score (TNS) and its variants (TNSc, TNSr) improve diagnostic fidelity by integrating symptoms, clinical signs (e.g., vibration loss, pinprick response, reflexes), and electrophysiology when available. These scores correlate with objective measures and facilitate longitudinal tracking of both motor and sensory deficits [50–52]. Patient-reported outcome measures (PROMs), including the EORTC QLQ-CIPN20 and the FACT/GOG-Ntx, assess neuropathy-related symptoms across sensory, motor, and autonomic domains [51]. Although useful for routine monitoring, they exhibit only moderate correlation with clinical and electrophysiological findings, reinforcing the need for multimodal integration. Objective bedside tools, such as tuning fork for vibration, monofilament testing for light touch, and pinprick or cold discrimination, provide low-cost methods to identify fiber-specific deficits. In particular, sensory testing in stocking-and-glove distribution offers early insights into length-dependent neuropathies, while handheld algometers may reveal mechanical hyperalgesia, albeit with reproducibility constraints [53]. Electrophysiological studies, especially nerve conduction studies (NCS), remain the gold standard for large-fiber assessment, particularly in platinum- and vinca-associated neuropathies [48, 54]. NCS enable early and subclinical detection of sensory neuropathies by measuring compound sensory and motor action potentials, with the sural and dorsal sural nerves being the most sensitive indicators of early dysfunction. Findings typically show a reduction in sensory action potential amplitude with preserved conduction velocities in cases of sensory neuronopathy, such as those induced by cisplatin and oxaliplatin, whereas a length-dependent axonal pattern predominates in taxane- or bortezomib-induced neuropathies. Despite their diagnostic value, NCS are limited to large fiber function and do not capture small fiber damage (Aδ and C fibers), necessitating complementary approaches such as quantitative sensory testing, skin biopsy, or advanced imaging modalities to fully characterize the spectrum of CIPN manifestations [55].

Over time, diagnostic profiles may shift. Among survivors more than 12-month post-chemotherapy, a majority exhibit entrapment syndromes or radiculopathies rather than classical polyneuropathy, suggesting evolving or misattributed symptomatology [55]. This highlights the importance of periodic reassessment in survivorship care. Emerging imaging modalities, including high-resolution ultrasound, magnetic resonance neurography, and diffusion tensor imaging, permit visualization of structural nerve damage and guide differential diagnosis, especially in suspected immune or radiation-induced syndromes [16].

In sum, clinical acumen must be supported by structured, fiber-informed assessment strategies. The integration of subjective and objective tools enables accurate diagnosis, stratification of intervention needs, and long-term tracking of neurofunctional outcomes.

5. Managing the unmanageable: Therapeutic pathways

5.1 Rethinking pharmacological strategies: Between evidence, practice, and mechanistic perspectives

The pharmacological management of TIPN presents a persistent mismatch between clinical trial evidence and its application in routine oncologic practice. While major oncology guidelines, including those from ASCO [19], NCCN [56], and ESMO [57], have established clear treatment recommendations, adherence remains inconsistent across institutions and clinical settings [10]. This gap reflects not only barriers related to clinician familiarity and systemic reimbursement policies but also the complexity of aligning therapeutic choices with patient-specific neurobiological profiles and symptom constellations.

Duloxetine remains the only agent with robust, guideline-supported efficacy in the treatment of painful CIPN. Its dual mechanism, serotonin and norepinephrine reuptake inhibition, modulates descending inhibitory pathways, mitigating central pain amplification. In the pivotal randomized controlled trial by Smith et al., duloxetine reduced pain severity by a clinically meaningful margin (−0.73 on a 0–10 scale), particularly among patients treated with oxaliplatin [58]. Subsequent meta-analyses have confirmed its superiority over placebo, leading ASCO, NCCN, and ESMO to endorse duloxetine as first-line pharmacotherapy, recommending a titration from 30 to 60 mg/day as tolerated [19, 56, 57]. Nonetheless, its real-world uptake remains limited: In a French national survey, fewer than 12% of oncologists reported routinely prescribing duloxetine for CIPN, instead favoring pregabalin or amitriptyline, agents with weaker evidence [10, 59]. The underutilization of duloxetine may stem from tolerability concerns (e.g., nausea, fatigue), a lack of clinician familiarity, or healthcare system constraints regarding off-label use and reimbursement.

Gabapentinoids, despite their popularity, have not demonstrated consistent benefit in controlled trials. Gabapentin and pregabalin act on the $\alpha 2\delta$ subunit of voltage-gated calcium channels to reduce neuronal excitability. Although widely prescribed, especially for neuropathic pain of mixed origin, meta-analyses indicate that their efficacy in CIPN is questionable [60]. A pooled analysis of eight RCTs ($n = 631$) found no significant improvement in average pain or functional outcomes, even when administered prophylactically. In therapeutic settings, pregabalin showed a non-significant trend toward reduced maximum pain (SMD −0.28), but failed to meet statistical thresholds. In the N00C3 trial, gabapentin did not outperform placebo [61], and head-to-head comparisons favor duloxetine in terms of symptom relief and emotional impact. Despite this, pregabalin remains among the most prescribed agents in France [10], reflecting a divergence between practice and evidence. Common adverse effects, sedation, cognitive slowing, and dizziness are generally mild, but clinically relevant in older adults. ASCO and NCCN discourage routine use of gabapentinoids, though ESMO allows for empirical use in cases involving coexisting insomnia or anxiety.

Tricyclic antidepressants (TCAs), including amitriptyline and nortriptyline, are often considered when duloxetine is contraindicated or unavailable [59]. Historically used for neuropathic pain, TCAs have not demonstrated clear efficacy in CIPN, and their anticholinergic burden raises concerns, particularly among older patients with cardiac comorbidities. For these reasons, ASCO advises against routine use, although ESMO suggests cautious use in patients with overlapping mood or sleep disturbances [19]. Venlafaxine has been explored primarily for its potential in preventing acute oxaliplatin-induced neuropathy. A randomized trial showed preventive benefits at 75 mg/day, likely due to serotonergic and noradrenergic modulation [62]. However, these findings have not been replicated at lower doses, and major guidelines do not currently endorse its use, underscoring the need for further validation. Topical pharmacological agents offer a mechanistically attractive option for localized neuropathic symptoms with minimal systemic side effects. Capsaicin 8% patches act on TRPV1-expressing C-fibers to induce reversible nociceptor defunctionalization [63]. Although not endorsed by ASCO or NCCN, ESMO recognizes capsaicin as a second-line option for localized, allodynic, or distal pain [56, 57]. Registry data suggest pain relief lasting up to 5 months following a single application [63]. Menthol 1% creams that target TRPM8 cold receptors have shown moderate promise in small proof-of-concept trials but lack RCT confirmation. Topical amitriptyline-ketamine-baclofen combinations and lidocaine 5% patches have not demonstrated efficacy over placebo in rigorous studies and are not recommended for routine use in CIPN by any oncology society.

Opioids, including tramadol, are reserved for cases of refractory pain with significant functional impairment, as they offer symptomatic relief but no disease-modifying effects [64]. Current ASCO guidelines emphasize that opioids should be considered only as a last resort due to their side effect profile and limited long-term benefit. Regarding cannabinoids, while their use among patients with cancer is rising, evidence remains limited. The 2024 ASCO guideline underscores that cannabis and cannabinoids should not be recommended for pain management or symptom palliation outside of clinical trials, except in the specific context of refractory chemotherapy-induced nausea and vomiting where they may be considered as adjuncts to standard antiemetic therapy [65].

Ultimately, while pharmacologic interventions remain a cornerstone in CIPN management, their application should be both evidence-informed and mechanistically aligned with the patient's clinical profile. In the absence of validated biomarkers to support a mechanistically stratified approach, decisions continue to rely on clinician expertise, patient tolerability, and pragmatic factors such as accessibility. As research advances, there is an urgent need for precision pharmacology guided by phenotyping, molecular diagnostics, and prospective biomarker validation to narrow the gap between therapeutic promise and clinical utility.

5.2 Non-pharmacological strategies: From mechanistic alignment to whole-person care

Non-pharmacological interventions are increasingly recognized as central components of a multimodal response to TIPN. Their appeal lies in their ability to address both pathophysiological mechanisms and contextual factors that pharmacologic approaches often fail to capture. Among these, peripheral cooling, physical exercise, neurostimulation, nutritional strategies, acupuncture, and behavioral interventions have each demonstrated varying levels of efficacy, offering complementary pathways toward symptom relief, functional improvement, and improved survivorship experience.

Cryotherapy has emerged as a promising, low-risk strategy to reduce the incidence and severity of taxane-induced neuropathy. The technique involves peripheral cooling of the hands and feet during chemotherapy infusion using frozen gloves, socks, or specialized cooling devices. Its primary mechanism is thought to be the induction of local vasoconstriction, which reduces drug perfusion in distal nerve beds and thereby minimizes neurotoxic exposure. A 2025 meta-analysis by Kumar et al. demonstrated that cryotherapy reduced the risk of grade ≥ 2 neuropathy by more than half (RR = 0.45, 95% CI: 0.27–0.77), with even stronger effects on motor and sensory domains (RR = 0.18–0.19). The intervention also led to a 76% reduction in severe neuropathy symptoms, as measured by the Patient Neurotoxicity Questionnaire [66]. These findings were corroborated by the POLAR trial [67], which directly compared cryotherapy with compression using surgical gloves. Both methods significantly reduced high-grade neuropathy, with cryotherapy producing a 21% absolute risk reduction and compression by a 14% reduction. Persistent benefit was observed at follow-up, suggesting durable neuroprotective effects [67]. Despite this, neither ASCO nor ESMO has yet endorsed cryotherapy or compression as standard preventive care, largely due to heterogeneity in cooling protocols and limited large-scale replication. Nonetheless, the benign safety profile, accessibility, and reproducibility of these methods position them as attractive options for individuals at heightened risk of CIPN, particularly when supported by informed consent and structured implementation.

Parallel to cryotherapy, exercise-based interventions offer a mechanistically grounded response to CIPN that transcends symptomatic relief. They are now regarded not merely as adjunctive, but as core therapeutic strategies, particularly in the context of rehabilitation. A growing body of high-quality evidence, including randomized trials and systematic reviews, supports their role in mitigating neuropathic symptoms, enhancing neuromuscular coordination, and improving quality of life. A systematic review by Knoerl et al. affirmed that multimodal exercise programs incorporating aerobic, strength, and balance components significantly reduce symptom severity, with sustained improvements in functional performance [68]. In a secondary analysis of a trial involving ovarian cancer patients, supervised exercise resulted in attenuated CIPN progression and improved balance and lower-limb function [69]. Tanay et al. reported similar benefits in mixed cohort of cancer patients following an 8-week multimodal program [38].

Mechanistically, exercise improves mitochondrial function, upregulates neurotrophic factors such as BDNF and NGF, and downregulates proinflammatory cytokines including IL-6, TNF-α, and IL-1β. It promotes synaptic remodeling and facilitates thalamocortical integration, contributing to improved sensory discrimination and reduced central sensitization. Sensorimotor retraining, including foot-ankle coordination and dynamic postural adjustment, directly targets proprioceptive impairments and fall risk, core deficits in large-fiber neuropathy [17]. Cao et al. further highlighted that combined aerobic and resistance programs yield the greatest functional benefits, although adherence and supervision remain critical determinants of success [46].

Neuromodulatory techniques, notably scrambler therapy (ST), represent another promising modality for refractory CIPN. Unlike traditional TENS, which primarily engages Aβ fibers, ST targets C-fiber input to reconfigure aberrant nociceptive processing through the delivery of "non-pain" electrical signals [70]. In a randomized controlled trial, 59% of patients receiving ST reported ≥50% symptom reduction, with sustained improvements noted in 38% at 10 weeks [71]. While the exact neurophysiological mechanisms remain to be fully elucidated, preliminary evidence suggests that ST induces central desensitization through modulation of dorsal horn and cortical pain networks. Despite the absence of formal guideline endorsement, the safety profile, ease of application, and consistent benefits observed in phase II trials make ST a candidate for integration into care pathways for patients with refractory or pain-dominant CIPN.

Acupuncture and electroacupuncture have also demonstrated efficacy in several randomized trials and meta-analyses. A recent umbrella review incorporating 14 systematic reviews found that acupuncture, including electroacupuncture and transcutaneous electrical acupoint stimulation (TEAS), improves nerve conduction velocity and reduces both subjective and objective measures of CIPN severity [72]. These effects are believed to result from modulation of endogenous opioid pathways, serotonergic and noradrenergic systems, and local cytokine signaling. The ACUCIN trial further confirmed that electroacupuncture enhances sensory function and pain control in patients treated with taxanes, though inconsistent findings in sham-controlled trials and variations in acupoint protocols temper definitive conclusions.

Nutritional interventions continue to generate interest due to their plausible biological relevance and potential scalability. Large observational studies consistently link poor dietary quality to increased neuropathy risk. Compton et al. [73] reported that colon cancer patients adhering to a diet rich in vegetables and low in processed meats had a significantly lower incidence of moderate-to-severe neuropathy. Similar findings were observed in studies by Knoerl et al. [74] and Compton et al. [73], where high scores on the Healthy Eating Index correlated with fewer CIPN-related functional limitations. Laboratory-based studies reinforce these observations: A systematic review by Brain et al. documented consistent associations between low serum vitamin D, hypomagnesemia, and hypoalbuminemia with increased CIPN severity, particularly in patients exposed to platinum agents [75].

Though supplementation with glutamine, omega-3 fatty acids, vitamin B complex, and acetyl-L-carnitine has shown mixed results, clinical guidelines currently discourage routine use due to concerns about chemotherapeutic interference and inconclusive efficacy [76]. For instance, trials involving acetyl-L-carnitine not only failed to demonstrate benefit but, in some cases, suggested potential exacerbation of neuropathic symptoms. Similarly, while glutamine and omega-3 fatty acids have shown promise in early-phase studies, data remain insufficient for clinical recommendations. Given these uncertainties, ASCO and ESMO emphasize a personalized, laboratory-informed approach, reserving supplementation for cases with documented deficiencies. In practice, the integration of nutritional support into oncology care should involve registered dietitians and be guided by metabolic profiling and ongoing symptom assessment.

Behavioral interventions and patient-centered education constitute the final pillar of a comprehensive CIPN strategy [38, 77, 78]. Evidence increasingly suggests that behavioral activation, symptom self-monitoring, and goal-directed feedback improve symptom disclosure, functional capacity, and treatment adherence. Many patients hesitate to report symptoms out of fear that oncologists will reduce chemotherapy dosage. This silence delays intervention and exacerbates morbidity. Structured behavioral programs that incorporate symptom diaries, feedback mechanisms, and digital coaching have demonstrated the improvements in neuropathic pain, functional outcomes, and patient empowerment. These interventions are most effective when grounded in theoretical models such as the Behavior Change Wheel and Normalization Process Theory and should be integrated into survivorship planning with institutional support.

Taken together, these diverse strategies illustrate the growing potential of non-pharmacological interventions in the management of CIPN. When implemented in an integrated, evidence-informed, and personalized manner, they address both the neurobiological underpinnings and the lived experiences of patients. Future directions should prioritize standardized protocols, mechanism-based targeting, and hybrid models that combine pharmacologic and non-pharmacologic approaches to optimize outcomes in this high-burden condition.

6. Radiation-induced peripheral neuropathy: Emerging complexity in a historically underestimated entity

RIPN represents a severe, yet frequently underrecognized, complication of cancer radiotherapy. It affects both somatic and autonomic nerves, with predominant involvement of the brachial and lumbosacral plexuses following high-dose regional irradiation, especially in breast, head and neck, and pelvic malignancies [79]. RIPN typically manifests months to decades after treatment; however, recent reports have identified acute, immune-mediated subtypes presenting within weeks post-exposure [16].

Mechanistically, chronic RIPN is dominated by progressive radiation-induced fibrosis (RIF), a process initiated by endothelial cell apoptosis and driven by TGF-β signaling, leading to activation of myofibroblasts and excessive extracellular matrix deposition [34, 80–82]. The resulting perineural fibrosis compresses nerve trunks, impairs oxygen diffusion, and promotes ischemic demyelination and axonal degeneration. Histopathological studies consistently demonstrate hyalinized vasculature, endoneurial thickening, and evidence of conduction block on neurophysiological testing [34, 79]. In contrast, early-onset RIPN may represent a distinct inflammatory-vascular entity. In a Mayo Clinic cohort study, patients developed painful monophasic sensorimotor deficits 2 to 5 months after radiotherapy. Biopsies revealed perivascular lymphocytic infiltration, microvasculitis, and hemosiderin-laden macrophages, suggesting an ischemic-infectious pathogenesis potentially responsive to corticosteroids [16]. This raises the prospect of a critical therapeutic window during which immunosuppressive treatment might attenuate or reverse evolving damage. Clinically, RIPN typically begins with numbness, paresthesia, and neuropathic pain, followed by progressive motor weakness. In advanced stages, patients may experience contractures secondary to perijoint fibrosis or complete flaccid paralysis coexisting with neuropathic pain [34]. Unlike tumor recurrence, which frequently presents with mass effect or infiltration, RIPN manifests with diffuse nerve thickening and T2-weighted hypointensity on MRI, reflecting fibrotic transformation rather than active inflammation [3, 16, 33]. Dosimetric thresholds play a decisive role in RIPN risk stratification. Involvement of the brachial or lumbosacral plexus is strongly associated with cumulative doses exceeding 50–60 Gy and fraction sizes >2 Gy [79]. Emerging evidence from stereotactic body radiation therapy (SBRT) protocols indicates that doses exceeding 40–45 Gy to the plexus, especially when overlapping major vessels or diabetic neurovasculature, may precipitate complications even in the absence of prior symptoms [82].

Management remains largely supportive. Neuropathic pain is addressed with anticonvulsants, tricyclic antidepressants, or corticosteroids in suspected inflammatory forms. Rehabilitation, including physiotherapy for joint preservation and functional maintenance, remains essential. In chronic fibrotic cases, surgical neurolysis may provide partial pain relief, although functional recovery remains limited: In one series, only 16–19% of patients experienced motor or sensory improvement postoperatively [34]. Experimental interventions are under exploration. Hyperbaric oxygen therapy has demonstrated some capacity to promote vascular repair and improve tissue oxygenation, though robust data remain scarce [33]. Preclinical work on mesenchymal stem cell transplantation has suggested potential for anti-fibrotic modulation and neuroregeneration, particularly in ischemic or fibrosclerotic nerve environments.

In summary, RIPN represents a complex and dynamic neuropathy encompassing both delayed fibrotic syndromes and acute inflammatory variants. Improved clinical awareness, adherence to precise dosimetric constraints, and the use of advanced imaging for early identification are essential to mitigate long-term disability.

7. Toward a personalized, multimodal algorithm

The translation of mechanistic insights into structured clinical decisions remains a persistent challenge in the management of TIPNs. While the underlying biological mechanisms of neurotoxicity have been increasingly clarified across oncologic treatments, there is still a striking lack of clinical tools capable of synthesizing these insights into personalized care strategies. In response, the present section proposes in **Figure 2** a decision support algorithm organized along three temporal

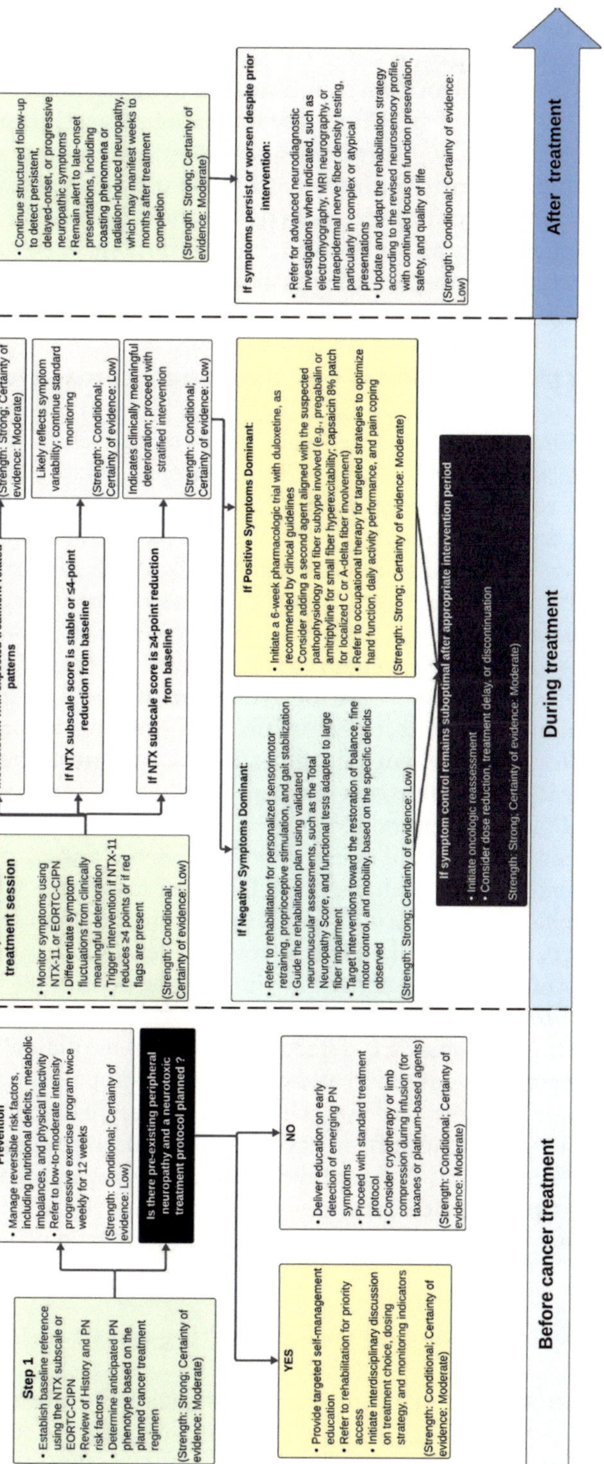

Figure 2.
Stratified algorithm for the monitoring and management of treatment-induced peripheral neuropathy.

phases: pre-treatment, treatment, and post-treatment. This model was developed to operationalize evidence-based knowledge into action-oriented recommendations, while accounting for fiber-specific symptom expression, neurotoxicity profiles of therapeutic classes, and patient-level vulnerability. Rather than imposing a prescriptive template, the algorithm functions as a flexible clinical framework. It integrates key components of stratified care including risk screening, symptom monitoring, treatment response thresholds, and intervention escalation, while remaining adaptable to interdisciplinary workflows and varied resource settings. Each phase corresponds to critical decision points that are explicitly linked to the timing and pathophysiology of TIPN onset, and to the clinical actions supported by the literature. To support transparent clinical reasoning, the certainty of evidence for each action has been indicated in the figure using GRADE-based labels.

7.1 Pre-treatment phase: Anchoring risk and planning proactively

Initial evaluation begins with the establishment of a baseline neurotoxicity profile using the NTX subscale or the EORTC-CIPN20. These validated instruments allow for quantification of pre-existing neuropathic symptoms, which is critical for detecting treatment-related deterioration later. The review of patient history should encompass comorbidities, prior neurotoxic exposures, and current risk factors, including nutritional deficits, metabolic derangements, or physical inactivity. At this stage, patients are stratified according to the presence or absence of pre-existing peripheral neuropathy, and whether a known neurotoxic protocol is planned. For individuals at increased risk, such as those with existing symptoms and an indication for platinum, taxane, or other high-risk agents, the algorithm recommends management of reversible risk factors, coupled with the initiation of a progressive exercise program over a 12-week period. This approach is based on evidence supporting the protective effects of prehabilitation on neural resilience and systemic inflammation. When neuropathy is already present and a neurotoxic regimen is anticipated, targeted self-management education should be provided prior to treatment initiation. Early referral to rehabilitation services is advised to ensure timely intervention. An interdisciplinary dialog should occur to review the suitability of the proposed protocol, dosing strategies, and monitoring indicators, potentially prompting dose modifications or alternative regimens.

If no pre-existing neuropathy is detected, clinicians should deliver education focused on early symptom detection and encourage prompt reporting of paresthesia, numbness, or motor changes. Patients scheduled to receive taxanes or platinum-based regimens may also benefit from cryotherapy or limb compression during infusion, which reduces local drug uptake and may lower peripheral nerve exposure. These interventions are particularly relevant in high-risk individuals and are supported by data demonstrating their feasibility, safety, and efficacy in selected populations.

7.2 Treatment phase: Threshold-based monitoring and stratified response

During active treatment, symptom monitoring should occur at every chemotherapy session. The NTX-11 or EORTC-CIPN questionnaires are recommended tools. Clinicians must distinguish between typical fluctuations and clinically meaningful deterioration. A $\geq$ four-point reduction on the NTX-11 subscale from baseline serves as a validated threshold for actionable change, correlating with reduced function and increased symptom burden. If symptoms remain stable or fluctuate within a four-point margin, continued routine monitoring is appropriate. In contrast, a ≥ four-point drop signals the need for stratified therapeutic intervention. The clinical trajectory is then guided by symptom typology. When negative sensory symptoms dominate—such as proprioceptive loss or impaired coordination, patients should be referred to rehabilitation for individualized sensorimotor retraining, balance restoration, and proprioceptive stimulation. Functional goals are shaped by validated neuromuscular assessments including the total neuropathy score, which helps identify large-fiber impairments requiring task-specific interventions. In patients with positive sensory symptoms—namely tingling, burning, or hyperalgesia, a 6-week pharmacologic trial with duloxetine should be initiated, in accordance with the current guidelines. If symptom control remains inadequate, adjunctive pharmacologic strategies may be considered. These should be matched to the suspected fiber subtype: pregabalin or amitriptyline for small-fiber hyperexcitability, or capsaicin 8% patches for localized symptoms suggestive of C or Aδ fiber involvement. Occupational therapy may be consulted to support hand function, daily activity performance, and pain self-management in cases of refractory symptoms.

When symptoms progress rapidly, occur independently of dosage, or present with a motor-predominant profile, urgent medical reassessment is warranted. Atypical, asymmetric, or inconsistent symptoms may reflect alternative diagnoses such as immune-mediated neuropathies. Referral to a neurologist should be considered to guide differential diagnosis and access specialized investigations. If, despite appropriate intervention, symptom control remains suboptimal, oncologic reassessment becomes necessary. Treatment decisions may involve reducing chemotherapy dose intensity, delaying administration, or discontinuing the regimen entirely. Such decisions should be made collaboratively, balancing oncologic efficacy against functional risk and patient preference.

7.3 Post-treatment phase: Longitudinal follow-up and functional recovery

Following the completion of neurotoxic treatment, the focus shifts toward structured follow-up to detect persistent, delayed-onset, or progressive neuropathy. Particular attention should be given to coasting phenomena, where symptoms worsen weeks after drug cessation, and radiation-induced neuropathies, which may manifest long after exposure. Surveillance should incorporate periodic reassessment using NTX-11 and composite tools such as TNSc or TNSr to monitor progression and inform treatment modification. In patients with unresolved or worsening symptoms, advanced diagnostics, including electromyography, MRI neurography, or intraepidermal nerve fiber density testing may be indicated to refine the neuropathy profile. Rehabilitation strategies should be revised based on updated findings, with a sustained emphasis on maintaining independence, preventing falls, and improving quality of life.

TIPN management should be fully embedded into survivorship care plans. This includes facilitating long-term access to physiotherapy, occupational therapy, pain management, and psychosocial support. Early integration of these services may mitigate the long-term consequences of peripheral nerve injury and optimize functional recovery throughout survivorship.

8. Conclusion

TIPN represents a significant clinical challenge at the intersection of oncology, neurology, and rehabilitation. This chapter has reviewed its diverse etiologies, phenotypic expressions, and current therapeutic options, highlighting both the limitations of existing pharmacological approaches and the emerging promise of non-pharmacological interventions. By integrating mechanistic knowledge, risk stratification, and phase-specific decision-making, the proposed algorithm offers a pragmatic framework for individualized care.

Moving forward, implementation of such structured pathways will require multidisciplinary coordination, improved symptom monitoring, and further validation across clinical contexts. Embedding TIPN management within survivorship care is essential to preserving functional autonomy, quality of life, and long-term treatment adherence in oncology populations.

Conflict of interest

The authors declare no conflict of interest.

Author details

Sébastien S. Dufresne[1,2,3]*, Pauline Jardel[4], Mélanie Brassard[4], Patricia Bilodeau[5] and Edith De Grand'Maison[5]

1 University of Quebec at Chicoutimi (UQAC), Saguenay, Canada

2 Intersectoral Center for Sustainable Health (CISD), Saguenay, Canada

3 Quebec Network for Research in Palliative and End-of-Life Care (RQSPAL), Quebec City, Canada

4 Integrated University Health and Social Services Centre of Saguenay–Lac-Saint-Jean (CIUSSS), Saguenay, Canada

5 Integrated Health and Social Services Centre of Chaudière-Appalaches (CISSS), Lévis, Canada

*Address all correspondence to: sebastien2_dufresne@uqac.ca

References

[1] Kerckhove N, Collin A, Conde S, et al. Chemotherapy-induced peripheral neuropathy: Symptomatology and epidemiology. Bulletin du Cancer. 2018;**105**:1020-1032. DOI: 10.1016/j.bulcan.2018.07.009

[2] Lavoie Smith EM, Von Ah D. Neurotoxicity in cancer survivorship: The significance of cancer-related cognitive impairment and chemotherapy-induced peripheral neuropathy. Seminars in Oncology Nursing. 2024;**40**:151724. DOI: 10.1016/j.soncn.2024.151724

[3] Harris SR. Brachial plexopathy after breast cancer: A persistent late effect of radiotherapy. PM & R : The Journal of Injury, Function, and Rehabilitation. 2024;**16**:85-91. DOI: 10.1002/pmrj.13007

[4] Colvin LA. Chemotherapy-induced peripheral neuropathy: Where are we now? Pain. 2019;**160**(Suppl. 1):S1-S10. DOI: 10.1097/j.pain.0000000000001540

[5] Seretny M, Currie GL, Sena ES, et al. Incidence, prevalence, and predictors of chemotherapy-induced peripheral neuropathy: A systematic review and meta-analysis. Pain. 2014;**155**:2461-2470. DOI: 10.1016/j.pain.2014.09.020

[6] Shah A, Hoffman EM, Mauermann ML, et al. Incidence and disease burden of chemotherapy-induced peripheral neuropathy in a population-based cohort. Journal of Neurology, Neurosurgery, and Psychiatry. 2018;**89**:636-641. DOI: 10.1136/jnnp-2017-317215

[7] van de Graaf DL, Engelen V, de Boer A, et al. Experiences of cancer survivors with chemotherapy-induced peripheral neuropathy in the Netherlands: Symptoms, daily limitations, involvement of healthcare professionals, and social support. Journal of Cancer Survivorship. 2024;**18**:1630-1639. DOI: 10.1007/s11764-023-01402-4

[8] Hershman DL, Till C, Wright JD, et al. Comorbidities and risk of chemotherapy-induced peripheral neuropathy among participants 65 years or older in southwest oncology group clinical trials. Journal of Clinical Oncology. 2016;**34**:3014-3022. DOI: 10.1200/JCO.2015.66.2346

[9] Mizrahi D, Park SB, Li T, et al. Hemoglobin, body mass index, and age as risk factors for paclitaxel- and oxaliplatin-induced peripheral neuropathy. JAMA Network Open. 2021;**4**:e2036695. DOI: 10.1001/jamanetworkopen.2020.36695

[10] Selvy M, Pereira B, Kerckhove N, et al. Prevention, diagnosis and management of chemotherapy-induced peripheral neuropathy: A cross-sectional study of French oncologists' professional practices. Support Care Cancer. 2021;**29**:4033-4043. DOI: 10.1007/s00520-020-05928-6

[11] Was H, Borkowska A, Bagues A, et al. Mechanisms of chemotherapy-induced neurotoxicity. Frontiers in Pharmacology. 2022;**13**:750507. DOI: 10.3389/fphar.2022.750507

[12] Malacrida A, Meregalli C, Rodriguez-Menendez V, et al. Chemotherapy-induced peripheral neuropathy and changes in cytoskeleton. International Journal of Molecular Sciences. 2019;**20**:2287. DOI: 10.3390/ijms20092287

[13] Trecarichi A, Flatters SJL. Mitochondrial dysfunction in the

pathogenesis of chemotherapy-induced peripheral neuropathy. International Review of Neurobiology. 2019;**145**:83-126. DOI: 10.1016/bs.irn.2019.05.001

[14] Mikami T, Liaw B, Asada M, et al. Neuroimmunological adverse events associated with immune checkpoint inhibitor: A retrospective, pharmacovigilance study using FAERS database. Journal of Neuro-Oncology. 2021;**152**:135-144. DOI: 10.1007/s11060-020-03687-2

[15] Ruggiero R, Balzano N, Di Napoli R, et al. Do peripheral neuropathies differ among immune checkpoint inhibitors? Reports from the European post-marketing surveillance database in the past 10 years. Frontiers in Immunology. 2023;**14**:1134436. DOI: 10.3389/fimmu.2023.1134436

[16] Skolka M, Shelly S, Pinto MV, et al. Clinical, neurophysiologic, and pathologic features in patients with early-onset postradiation neuropathy. Neurology. 2023;**101**:e1455-e1460. DOI: 10.1212/WNL.0000000000207545

[17] Stoller S, Capozza S, Alberti P, et al. Framework to leverage physical therapists for the assessment and treatment of chemotherapy-induced peripheral neurotoxicity (CIPN). Support Care Cancer. 2023;**31**:293. DOI: 10.1007/s00520-023-07734-2

[18] Hertz DL, Childs DS, Park SB, et al. Patient-centric decision framework for treatment alterations in patients with chemotherapy-induced peripheral neuropathy (CIPN). Cancer Treatment Reviews. 2021;**99**:102241. DOI: 10.1016/j.ctrv.2021.102241

[19] Loprinzi CL, Lacchetti C, Bleeker J, et al. Prevention and management of chemotherapy-induced peripheral neuropathy in survivors of adult cancers: ASCO guideline update. Journal of Clinical Oncology. 2020;**38**:3325-3348. DOI: 10.1200/JCO.20.01399

[20] Molassiotis A, Cheng HL, Leung KT, et al. Risk factors for chemotherapy-induced peripheral neuropathy in patients receiving taxane- and platinum-based chemotherapy. Brain and Behavior: A Cognitive Neuroscience Perspective. 2019;**9**:e01312. DOI: 10.1002/brb3.1312

[21] Mizrahi D, Goldstein D, Kiernan MC, et al. Development and consensus process for a clinical pathway for the assessment and management of chemotherapy-induced peripheral neuropathy. Support Care Cancer. 2022;**30**:5965-5974. DOI: 10.1007/s00520-022-07024-3

[22] Li Y, Marri T, North RY, et al. Chemotherapy-induced peripheral neuropathy in a dish: Dorsal root ganglion cells treated in vitro with paclitaxel show biochemical and physiological responses parallel to that seen in vivo. Pain. 2021;**162**:84-96. DOI: 10.1097/j.pain.0000000000002005

[23] Best RL, LaPointe NE, Azarenko O, et al. Microtubule and tubulin binding and regulation of microtubule dynamics by the antibody drug conjugate (ADC) payload, monomethyl auristatin E (MMAE): Mechanistic insights into MMAE ADC peripheral neuropathy. Toxicology and Applied Pharmacology. 2021;**421**:115534. DOI: 10.1016/j.taap.2021.115534

[24] Cartelli D, Cavaletti G, Lauria G, et al. Ubiquitin proteasome system and microtubules are master regulators of central and peripheral nervous system axon degeneration. Cells. 2022;**11**. DOI: 10.3390/cells11081358

[25] Yang Y, Zhao B, Gao X, et al. Targeting strategies for

oxaliplatin-induced peripheral neuropathy: Clinical syndrome, molecular basis, and drug development. Journal of Experimental & Clinical Cancer Research. 2021;**40**:331. DOI: 10.1186/s13046-021-02141-z

[26] Pinheiro EA, Magdy T, Burridge PW. Human in vitro models for assessing the genomic basis of chemotherapy-induced cardiovascular toxicity. Journal of Cardiovascular Translational Research. 2020;**13**:377-389. DOI: 10.1007/s12265-020-09962-x

[27] Kang L, Tian Y, Xu S, et al. Oxaliplatin-induced peripheral neuropathy: Clinical features, mechanisms, prevention and treatment. Journal of Neurology. 2021;**268**:3269-3282. DOI: 10.1007/s00415-020-09942-w

[28] Li Y, Lustberg MB, Hu S. Emerging pharmacological and non-pharmacological therapeutics for prevention and treatment of chemotherapy-induced peripheral neuropathy. Cancers (Basel). 2021;**13**. DOI: 10.3390/cancers13040766

[29] Lee JH, Kim W. The role of satellite glial cells, astrocytes, and microglia in oxaliplatin-induced neuropathic pain. Biomedicine. 2020;**8**. DOI: 10.3390/biomedicines8090324

[30] Johnson DB, Manouchehri A, Haugh AM, et al. Neurologic toxicity associated with immune checkpoint inhibitors: A pharmacovigilance study. Journal for Immunotherapy of Cancer. 2019;**7**:134. DOI: 10.1186/s40425-019-0617-x

[31] Fu Z, Gao C, Wu T, et al. Peripheral neuropathy associated with monomethyl auristatin E-based antibody-drug conjugates. iScience. 2023;**26**:107778. DOI: 10.1016/j.isci.2023.107778

[32] Diez P, Hanna GG, Aitken KL, et al. UK 2022 consensus on normal tissue dose-volume constraints for oligometastatic, primary lung and hepatocellular carcinoma stereotactic ablative radiotherapy. Clinical Oncology (Royal College of Radiologists). 2022;**34**:288-300. DOI: 10.1016/j.clon.2022.02.010

[33] Milano MT, Mavroidis P, Ryckman J, et al. Radiation-induced inferior brachial plexopathy after stereotactic body radiotherapy: Pooled analyses of risks. Radiotherapy and Oncology. 2023;**182**:109583. DOI: 10.1016/j.radonc.2023.109583

[34] Shekouhi R, Gerhold C, Chim H. The role of surgery in the management of radiation-induced brachial plexopathy: A systematic review. Journal of Hand Surgery (European Volume). 2024;**49**:490-498. DOI: 10.1177/17531934231197794

[35] Lee KT, Bulls HW, Hoogland AI, et al. Chemotherapy-induced peripheral neuropathy (CIPN): A narrative review and proposed theoretical model. Cancers (Basel). 2024;**16**. DOI: 10.3390/cancers16142571

[36] Barakat HE, Hussein RRS, Elberry AA, et al. The impact of metformin use on the outcomes of locally advanced breast cancer patients receiving neoadjuvant chemotherapy: An open-labelled randomized controlled trial. Scientific Reports. 2022;**12**:7656. DOI: 10.1038/s41598-022-11138-3

[37] Hershey DS. Importance of glycemic control in cancer patients with diabetes: Treatment through end of life. Asia-Pacific Journal of Oncology Nursing. 2017;**4**:313-318. DOI: 10.4103/apjon.apjon_40_17

[38] Tanay MAL, Armes J, Moss-Morris R, et al. A systematic review of

behavioural and exercise interventions for the prevention and management of chemotherapy-induced peripheral neuropathy symptoms. Journal of Cancer Survivorship. 2023;**17**:254-277. DOI: 10.1007/s11764-021-00997-w

[39] El-Najjar SE, Naser IA, Al-Wahidi KM. Is functional vitamin B12 deficiency a risk factor for the development of chemotherapy-induced peripheral neuropathy in cancer patients? Asian Pacific Journal of Cancer Prevention. 2025;**26**:375-382. DOI: 10.31557/APJCP.2025.26.2.375

[40] Frediani JK, Lal AA, Kim E, et al. The role of diet and non-pharmacologic supplements in the treatment of chronic neuropathic pain: A systematic review. Pain Practice. 2024;**24**:186-210. DOI: 10.1111/papr.13291

[41] Tofthagen C, Tanay M, Perlman A, et al. A systematic review of nutritional lab correlates with chemotherapy induced peripheral neuropathy. Journal of Clinical Medicine. 2022;**11**. DOI: 10.3390/jcm11020355

[42] Wesselink E, Winkels RM, van Baar H, et al. Dietary intake of magnesium or calcium and chemotherapy-induced peripheral neuropathy in colorectal cancer patients. Nutrients. 2018;**10**. DOI: 10.3390/nu10040398

[43] Bjornard KL, Gilchrist LS, Inaba H, et al. Peripheral neuropathy in children and adolescents treated for cancer. The Lancet Child & Adolescent Health. 2018;**2**:744-754. DOI: 10.1016/S2352-4642(18)30236-0

[44] Sanchez-Barroso L, Apellaniz-Ruiz M, Gutierrez-Gutierrez G, et al. Concomitant medications and risk of chemotherapy-induced peripheral neuropathy. The Oncologist. 2019;**24**:e784-e792. DOI: 10.1634/theoncologist.2018-0418

[45] Timmins HC, Mizrahi D, Li T, et al. Metabolic and lifestyle risk factors for chemotherapy-induced peripheral neuropathy in taxane and platinum-treated patients: A systematic review. Journal of Cancer Survivorship. 2023;**17**:222-236. DOI: 10.1007/s11764-021-00988-x

[46] Cao A, Cartmel B, Li FY, et al. Effect of exercise on chemotherapy-induced peripheral neuropathy among patients treated for ovarian cancer: A secondary analysis of a randomized clinical trial. JAMA Network Open. 2023;**6**:e2326463. DOI: 10.1001/jamanetworkopen.2023.26463

[47] Relias V, Maloney A, Smith MH, et al. Does "OPTINAB" strategy ("stop-and-go") work in treatment of advanced pancreatic cancer (APC) with nab-paclitaxel-gemcitabine? Cancer Chemotherapy and Pharmacology. 2017;**80**:371-375. DOI: 10.1007/s00280-017-3374-x

[48] Molassiotis A, Cheng HL, Lopez V, et al. Are we mis-estimating chemotherapy-induced peripheral neuropathy? Analysis of assessment methodologies from a prospective, multinational, longitudinal cohort study of patients receiving neurotoxic chemotherapy. BMC Cancer. 2019;**19**:132. DOI: 10.1186/s12885-019-5302-4

[49] Ogle T, Alexander K, Miaskowski C, et al. Systematic review of the effectiveness of self-initiated interventions to decrease pain and sensory disturbances associated with peripheral neuropathy. Journal of Cancer Survivorship. 2020;**14**:444-463. DOI: 10.1007/s11764-020-00861-3

[50] Belloni S, Magon A, Giacon C, et al. Peripheral neuropathy instruments for individuals with cancer: A COSMIN-based systematic review of measurement properties. Current Oncology. 2024;**31**:7828-7851. DOI: 10.3390/curroncol31120577

[51] Li T, Park SB, Battaglini E, et al. Assessing chemotherapy-induced peripheral neuropathy with patient reported outcome measures: A systematic review of measurement properties and considerations for future use. Quality of Life Research. 2022;**31**:3091-3107. DOI: 10.1007/s11136-022-03154-7

[52] Song SY, Park JH, Lee JS, et al. A randomized, placebo-controlled trial evaluating changes in peripheral neuropathy and quality of life by using low-frequency electrostimulation on breast cancer patients treated with chemotherapy. Integrative Cancer Therapies. 2020;**19**:1534735420925519. DOI: 10.1177/1534735420925519

[53] Stubblefield MD, McNeely ML, Alfano CM, et al. A prospective surveillance model for physical rehabilitation of women with breast cancer: Chemotherapy-induced peripheral neuropathy. Cancer. 2012;**118**:2250-2260. DOI: 10.1002/cncr.27463

[54] Taoka R, Kamada M, Izumi K, et al. Peripheral neuropathy and nerve electrophysiological changes with enfortumab vedotin in patients with advanced urothelial carcinoma: A prospective multicenter cohort study. International Journal of Clinical Oncology. 2024;**29**:602-611. DOI: 10.1007/s10147-024-02481-8

[55] Argyriou AA, Park SB, Islam B, et al. Neurophysiological, nerve imaging and other techniques to assess chemotherapy-induced peripheral neurotoxicity in the clinical and research settings. Journal of Neurology, Neurosurgery, and Psychiatry. 2019;**90**:1361-1369. DOI: 10.1136/jnnp-2019-320969

[56] Swarm RA, Paice JA, Anghelescu DL, et al. Adult cancer pain, version 3.2019, NCCN clinical practice guidelines in oncology. Journal of the National Comprehensive Cancer Network. 2019;**17**:977-1007. DOI: 10.6004/jnccn.2019.0038

[57] Jordan B, Margulies A, Cardoso F, et al. Systemic anticancer therapy-induced peripheral and central neurotoxicity: ESMO-EONS-EANO clinical practice guidelines for diagnosis, prevention, treatment and follow-up. Annals of Oncology. 2020;**31**:1306-1319. DOI: 10.1016/j.annonc.2020.07.003

[58] Smith EM, Pang H, Cirrincione C, et al. Effect of duloxetine on pain, function, and quality of life among patients with chemotherapy-induced painful peripheral neuropathy: A randomized clinical trial. JAMA. 2013;**309**:1359-1367. DOI: 10.1001/jama.2013.2813

[59] Moisset X, Bouhassira D, Avez Couturier J, et al. Pharmacological and non-pharmacological treatments for neuropathic pain: Systematic review and French recommendations. Revue Neurologique (Paris). 2020;**176**:325-352. DOI: 10.1016/j.neurol.2020.01.361

[60] Chang TW, Yang FY, Liu YC, et al. Gabapentinoids for chemotherapy-induced peripheral neuropathy: Systematic review and meta-analysis. BMJ Supportive & Palliative Care. 2024;**14**:269-278. DOI: 10.1136/spcare-2023-004362

[61] Rao RD, Michalak JC, Sloan JA, et al. Efficacy of gabapentin in the management of chemotherapy-induced

peripheral neuropathy: A phase 3 randomized, double-blind, placebo-controlled, crossover trial (N00C3). Cancer. 2007;**110**:2110-2118. DOI: 10.1002/cncr.23008

[62] Durand JP, Deplanque G, Montheil V, et al. Efficacy of venlafaxine for the prevention and relief of oxaliplatin-induced acute neurotoxicity: Results of EFFOX, a randomized, double-blind, placebo-controlled phase III trial. Annals of Oncology. 2012;**23**:200-205. DOI: 10.1093/annonc/mdr045

[63] Maihofner C, Diel I, Tesch H, et al. Chemotherapy-induced peripheral neuropathy (CIPN): Current therapies and topical treatment option with high-concentration capsaicin. Support Care Cancer. 2021;**29**:4223-4238. DOI: 10.1007/s00520-021-06042-x

[64] Glare P, Aubrey K, Gulati A, et al. Pharmacologic management of persistent pain in cancer survivors. Drugs. 2022;**82**:275-291. DOI: 10.1007/s40265-022-01675-6

[65] Braun IM, Bohlke K, Abrams DI, et al. Cannabis and cannabinoids in adults with cancer: ASCO guideline. Journal of Clinical Oncology. 2024;**42**:1575-1593. DOI: 10.1200/JCO.23.02596

[66] Ashok Kumar P, Sampat P, Sandhu M, et al. A meta-analysis of the utility of cryotherapy for preventing peripheral neuropathy among breast cancer patients receiving paclitaxel and nab-paclitaxel. Breast Cancer Research and Treatment. 2025;**210**:595-604. DOI: 10.1007/s10549-024-07597-z

[67] Michel LL, Schwarz D, Romar P, et al. Efficacy of hand cooling and compression in preventing taxane-induced neuropathy: The POLAR randomized clinical trial. JAMA Oncology. 2025;**11**:408-415. DOI: 10.1001/jamaoncol.2025.0001

[68] Knoerl R, Gilchrist L, Kanzawa-Lee GA, et al. Proactive rehabilitation for chemotherapy-induced peripheral neuropathy. Seminars in Oncology Nursing. 2020;**36**:150983. DOI: 10.1016/j.soncn.2019.150983

[69] Kleckner IR, Park SB, Streckmann F, Wiskemann J, Hardy S, Mohile N. Clinical and practical recommendations in the use of exercise, physical therapy, and occupational therapy for chemotherapy-induced peripheral neuropathy. In: Lustberg M, Loprinzi C, editors. Diagnosis, Management and Emerging Strategies for Chemotherapy-Induced Neuropathy. Cham, Switzerland: Springer; 2021. pp. 183-241. DOI: 10.1007/978-3-030-78663-2_9

[70] D'Souza RS, Her YF, Jin MY, et al. Neuromodulation therapy for chemotherapy-induced peripheral neuropathy: A systematic review. Biomedicine. 2022;**10**. DOI: 10.3390/biomedicines10081909

[71] Loprinzi C, Le-Rademacher JG, Majithia N, et al. Scrambler therapy for chemotherapy neuropathy: A randomized phase II pilot trial. Support Care Cancer. 2020;**28**:1183-1197. DOI: 10.1007/s00520-019-04881-3

[72] Klafke N, Bossert J, Kroger B, et al. Prevention and treatment of chemotherapy-induced peripheral neuropathy (CIPN) with non-pharmacological interventions: Clinical recommendations from a systematic scoping review and an expert consensus process. Medical Sciences. 2023;**11**. DOI: 10.3390/medsci11010015

[73] Compton SLE, Yang S, Madere J, et al. Dietary quality and chemotherapy-induced peripheral neuropathy in

colon cancer. Cancer. 2025;**131**:e35599. DOI: 10.1002/cncr.35599

[74] Knoerl R, Ploutz-Snyder R, Smener L, et al. Association of chemotherapy-induced peripheral neuropathy with diet quality among post-treatment cancer survivors. Nutrition and Cancer. 2024;**76**:717-725. DOI: 10.1080/01635581.2024.2364389

[75] Brain K, Burrows TL, Rollo ME, et al. A systematic review and meta-analysis of nutrition interventions for chronic noncancer pain. Journal of Human Nutrition and Dietetics. 2019;**32**:198-225. DOI: 10.1111/jhn.12601

[76] Giridhar KV, Viscuse PV, Loprinzi CL, et al. Supplements to help prevent neuropathy during chemotherapy? A cautionary tale. Journal of the National Cancer Institute. 2018;**110**:551-552. DOI: 10.1093/jnci/djx294

[77] Nyrop KA, Deal AM, Reeder-Hayes KE, et al. Patient-reported and clinician-reported chemotherapy-induced peripheral neuropathy in patients with early breast cancer: Current clinical practice. Cancer. 2019;**125**:2945-2954. DOI: 10.1002/cncr.32175

[78] van de Graaf DL, Mols F, Smeets T, et al. Coping with and self-management of chronic painful chemotherapy-induced peripheral neuropathy: A qualitative study among cancer survivors. Journal of Cancer Survivorship. 2025;**19**:295-305. DOI: 10.1007/s11764-023-01466-2

[79] Warade AC, Jha AK, Pattankar S, et al. Radiation-induced brachial plexus neuropathy: A review. Neurology India. 2019;**67**:S47-S52. DOI: 10.4103/0028-3886.250704

[80] Miran C, Bonnet E, Lafont C, et al. Radiation induced brachial plexopathy: Diagnosis, risk factors, principles of care. Cancer Radiothérapie. 2023;**27**:163-169. DOI: 10.1016/j.canrad.2022.06.010

[81] Verginadis II, Citrin DE, Ky B, et al. Radiotherapy toxicities: Mechanisms, management, and future directions. Lancet. 2025;**405**:338-352. DOI: 10.1016/S0140-6736(24)02319-5

[82] Wei JY, Ma LX, Liu WT, et al. Mechanisms and protective measures for radiation-induced brachial plexus nerve injury. Brain Research Bulletin. 2024;**210**:110924. DOI: 10.1016/j.brainresbull.2024.110924

Section 5

General Insights and Perspectives

Chapter 5

Insights into Peripheral Neuropathy

Hafsa Ahsan, Wajida Perveen, Asma Hussain and Sahreen Anwar

Abstract

Peripheral neuropathy is a heterogeneous disorder characterized by injury to the peripheral nerves, which may lead to many sensory, motor, autonomic, or a combination of any of the symptoms. The clinical presentation of peripheral neuropathy includes sensory impairments such as numbness, tingling, burning pain, and hypersensitivity, predominantly affecting the distal extremities. Motor impairments, including weakness, muscle atrophy, and impaired coordination, may also occur, which causes activity limitations and participation restrictions. Additionally, autonomic dysfunction causes further complications such as gastrointestinal disturbances, orthostatic hypotension, and urinary retention. These symptoms can range from mild to severe pain and disability, ultimately impacting the quality of life of the suffering individuals. This chapter is based on an overview of the etiology, pathophysiology, and treatment options of peripheral neuropathy.

Keywords: peripheral neuropathy, sensory neuropathy, motor neuropathy, autonomic neuropathy, diabetic neuropathy

1. Introduction

Any condition affecting the peripheral nervous system is referred to as peripheral neuropathy, including symmetrical involvement of polyneuropathy and asymmetric mononeuropathy [1, 2]. It is a heterogeneous disorder that is characterized by injury to the peripheral nerves, which leads to many sensory, motor, and autonomic symptoms. These symptoms can range from mild to severe pain and disability, ultimately impacting the quality of life for those who are impacted. The sensory loss occurs in a "glove and stocking" manner because of distal symmetric sensorimotor polyneuropathy, which is the most prevalent type of peripheral neuropathy [3]. However, its incidence is expected to rise with an aging population and cause conditions such as diabetes mellitus, autoimmune diseases, and cancer [4]. A study conducted in 2024 by Perveen W. et al. shows that using the Michigan Neuropathy Screening Instrument, the prevalence of peripheral neuropathy was 44.4 and 51.1%, respectively, based on a self-administered questionnaire and foot examination [3].

Various underlying causes lead toward the development of metabolic disorders, inflammatory conditions, infections, toxic exposures, and genetic predispositions because of the multifactorial nature of peripheral neuropathy [4]. The pathophysiology of peripheral neuropathy is complex, involving mechanisms such as neuronal damage,

IntechOpen

demyelination, inflammation, and impaired nerve regeneration. Peripheral nerve injury exhibits a pattern of segmental demyelination, which consists of the myelin sheath degenerating while the nerve axon remains intact. Mononeuropathies, sensorimotor disorders, and primarily motor neuropathies can all exhibit this kind of response. These are occasionally immune-mediated and frequently inflammatory. Myelin injury accounts for about 20% of symmetrical peripheral neuropathies. Examples include neuropathy linked to monoclonal gammopathy of unknown relevance and Charcot-Marie-Tooth disease. When a nerve axon degenerates as a result of a lesion or physical compression, the part distal to the axon passively wastes away, most likely because the cell body is not providing enough nutrition. This is known as Wallerian degeneration. Within 3 to 5 hours following the absence of spontaneous end-plate potentials, normal end-plate structures change. Focal mononeuropathy, which is secondary to nerve damage or infarction, is the outcome of this reaction. Axonal degeneration is a "dying-back" phenomenon, where axons degenerate in a distal to proximal manner, causing symmetrical polyneuropathy in 80% of cases. The mechanism is that a calcium-dependent cytoskeletal breakdown can occur as a result of a nerve injury that impairs the delivery of local axonal survival factors, raising intra-axonal calcium levels. Axonal degeneration can result from several illnesses, such as Guillain-Barre syndrome, diabetes, HIV, and the hepatitis C virus [5–7]. The clinical presentation of peripheral neuropathy includes sensory impairments such as numbness, tingling, burning pain, and hypersensitivity, predominantly affecting the distal extremities. Motor impairments, including weakness, muscle atrophy, and impaired coordination, may also occur, which causes activity limitations and participation restrictions. Additionally, autonomic dysfunction causes further complications such as gastrointestinal disturbances, orthostatic hypotension, and urinary retention [4]. Further neuropathy complications result in infection, ulcer, or even amputation, which has an adverse effect on quality of life in relation to health [3]. Diagnosing peripheral neuropathy requires clinical evaluation, neurophysiological testing, imaging studies, and laboratory investigations. History and the physical examination focused on the onset of the symptoms, their distribution, progression, and the risk factors that are associated with them [8].

Management of peripheral neuropathy is quite challenging, and it is usually based on clinical manifestations. The ultimate goal of the treatment is to alleviate impairments and improve functional status and quality of life. Pharmacological interventions such as analgesics, antidepressants, and topical agents are frequently utilized to manage pain and sensory impairments [9]. Non-pharmacological interventions such as physical therapy, including electrotherapy, therapeutic exercises, and manual therapy, may enhance muscle strength, mobility, and coordination. Lifestyle modifications such as smoking cessation, dietary changes, and regular physical activity are beneficial in combating the risk factors and for managing the symptoms caused by peripheral neuropathy (**Figure 1**) [4].

1.1 Etiology of peripheral neuropathy

Because of the multifactorial nature of peripheral neuropathy, understanding the etiological factors is crucial for making the diagnosis and appropriate treatment plan. The following are the etiological factors of peripheral neuropathy:

1. Diabetes mellitus

2. Chronic alcoholism

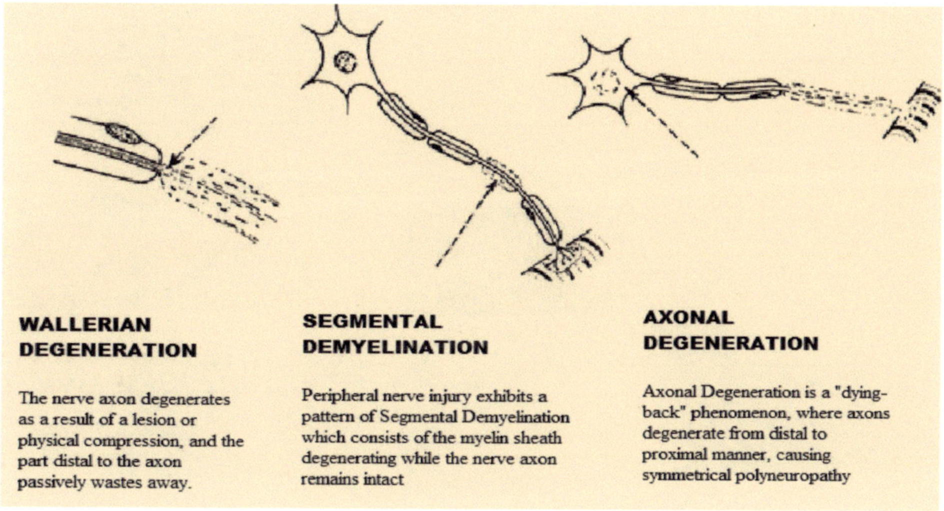

Figure 1.
Wallerian degeneration, segmental demyelination, and axonal degeneration.

3. Injury or trauma

4. Nutritional deficiencies (e.g., B1, B6, B12, and vitamin E)

5. Vascular Disorders (e.g., vasculitis)

6. Metabolic Disorders (e.g., uremia, hypothyroidism)

7. Infections (e.g., Lyme disease, Epstein-Barr virus, hepatitis C, shingles, leprosy, HIV)

8. Toxins (heavy metals, chemicals)

9. Chemotherapy agents

10. Medications (antibiotics, cardiovascular medications)

11. Tumors (secondary to compression or associated paraneoplastic syndromes)

12. Autoimmune disease (e.g., rheumatoid arthritis and Guillain-Barre syndrome)

13. Genetic predispositions (e.g., Charcot-Marie-Tooth disease) (**Figure 2**)

Diabetes mellitus: It is one of the main causes of peripheral neuropathy worldwide. Prolonged hyperglycemia induces microvascular alterations and metabolic disturbances that result in nerve damage. Reduced neuronal blood supply, inflammatory pathway activation, and the production of advanced glycation end products are some of the underlying processes [10]. Diabetic peripheral neuropathy is marked by two major clinical manifestations: neuropathic pain and diabetic foot ulceration. It is a leading cause of lower-limb amputation, significantly affecting the quality of life of those impacted [3].

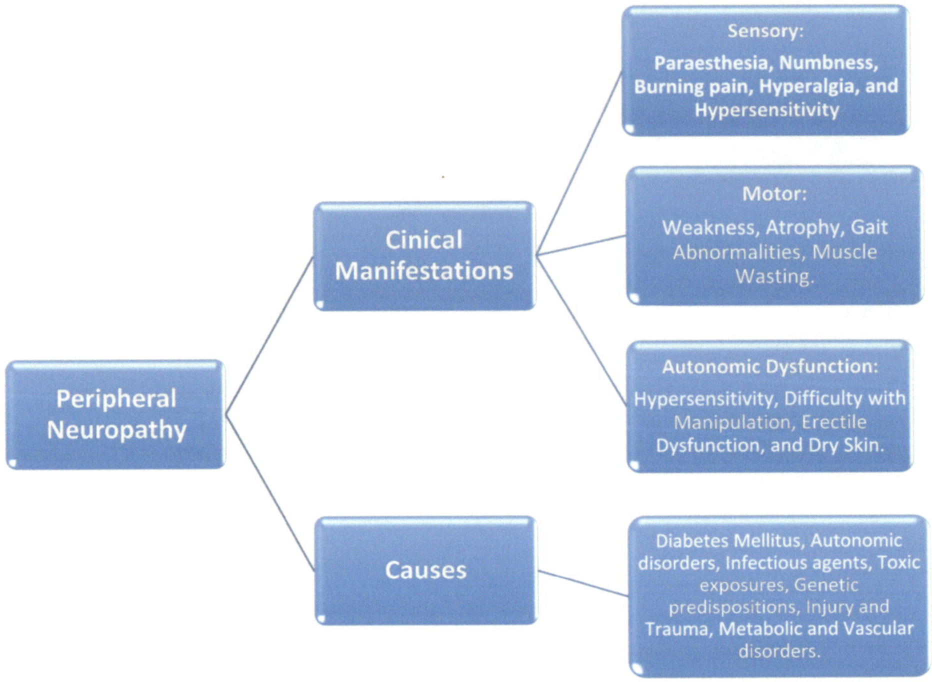

Figure 2.
Clinical manifestations and causes of the peripheral neuropathy.

Autoimmune disorders: Guillain-Barré syndrome (GBS), chronic inflammatory demyelinating polyneuropathy (CIDP), Sjögren's syndrome, and rheumatoid arthritis are examples of autoimmune illnesses that contribute significantly to peripheral neuropathy cases. In conditions like GBS and CIDP, abnormal immune responses attack peripheral nerve components, causing demyelination and axonal damage. Clinical manifestations vary by condition but commonly include progressive weakness, sensory impairments, and autonomic dysfunction [11].

Infectious agents: Peripheral neuropathy can result from various infectious agents through direct nerve invasion, immune-mediated processes, or toxin production. Notable examples include bacterial infections like Lyme disease and leprosy, as well as viruses like cytomegalovirus, human immunodeficiency virus, varicella-zoster virus, and herpes simplex virus. These pathogens cause neuronal damage, triggering inflammatory responses. Clinical presentations range from acute mononeuropathies to chronic polyneuropathies, encompassing a wide array of sensory, motor, and autonomic symptoms [12].

Toxic exposures: Peripheral neuropathy can result from exposure to neurotoxic substances, including alcohol, chemotherapeutic agents, heavy metals, industrial solvents, and certain medications. These toxins impair nerve structure and function through mechanisms such as oxidative stress, mitochondrial dysfunction, and disruption of neurotransmitter signaling. Symptoms typically include sensory disturbances, motor weakness, and neuropathic pain, with the clinical presentation varying based on the specific toxin and level of exposure [4].

Genetic predispositions: Hereditary neuropathies, caused by genetic mutations affecting nerve structure and function, comprise ailments such as familial amyloid polyneuropathy, hereditary sensory and autonomic neuropathies, and

Charcot-Marie-Tooth syndrome. These disorders present with varied clinical features, including distal muscle wasting, sensory deficits, and autonomic dysfunction. Genetic testing is essential for accurate diagnosis and managing these conditions [4].

Injury or trauma: Serious nerve damage can result from physical trauma or injury, including falls, automobile accidents, sports, and medical operations. A study conducted in 2021 by Perveen W. et al. presented a case report of an upper limb tourniquet palsy where the radial, ulnar, and median nerves were affected during surgery. It is a rare side effect of orthopedic surgery, and physical therapy is one of the promising forms of therapy for a full recovery, preventing impairment and returning to work [13].

Metabolic disorders: Metabolic abnormalities, such as vitamin deficiencies (e.g., B12, thiamine), uremia, and hypothyroidism, can cause peripheral neuropathy by disrupting nerve metabolism and myelin synthesis. These imbalances impair nerve conduction and maintenance, leading to sensory, motor, and autonomic dysfunction. Early identification and correction of the underlying metabolic issues are crucial for effectively managing neuropathy linked to these conditions [14].

Vascular disorders: Peripheral neuropathy can develop secondary to vascular insufficiency in conditions like peripheral artery disease and vasculitis. This deprivation of oxygen and nutrients leads to nerve dysfunction, with symptoms such as intermittent claudication, rest pain, and sensory deficits in affected areas. Treatment aims to enhance vascular perfusion through lifestyle changes, pharmacotherapy, or surgical interventions to relieve ischemic neuropathy symptoms [4].

Other causes: Peripheral neuropathy can be associated with neoplastic disorders, paraneoplastic syndromes, and connective tissue diseases. Rheumatoid arthritis and systemic lupus erythematosus (SLE) are examples of connective tissue diseases that may cause neuropathies through immune-mediated mechanisms (**Figure 3**) [15].

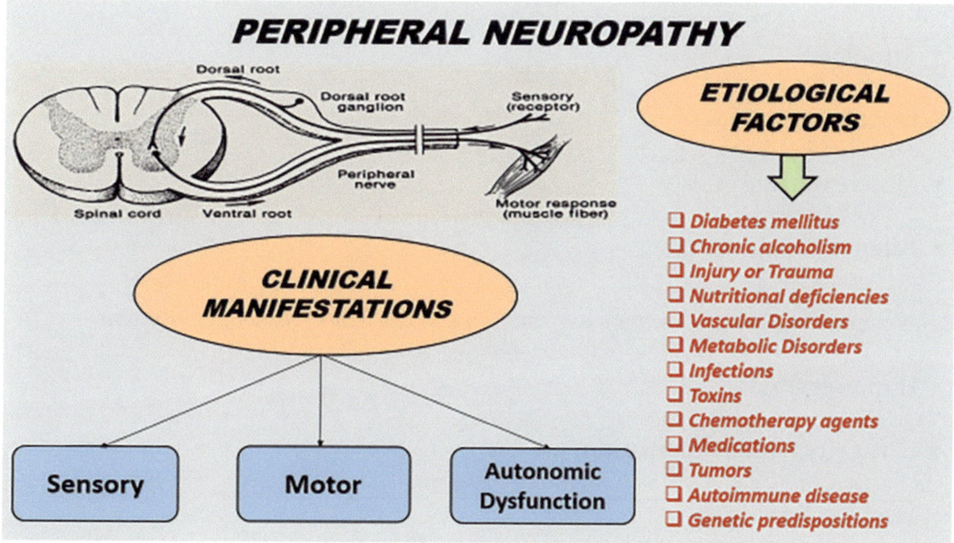

Figure 3.
Clinical manifestation and etiological factors of peripheral neuropathy.

1.2 Clinical manifestations of peripheral neuropathies

Peripheral neuropathy symptoms are rarely fatal; however, they can vary from mild to severe. The kind and extent of injury, as well as the kind of nerve fibers impacted, determine the symptoms. Over the course of days, weeks, or years, symptoms may appear. Sometimes, the symptoms go away on their own and do not need any special attention or care. Pain is a common symptom of peripheral neuropathy. Sometimes, neuropathic pain is more severe at night, which interferes with sleep. It can be brought on by pain receptors firing on their own without any recognized cause or by issues with the spinal cord's signal processing, which can result in excruciating pain from a typically light touch. We refer to this as allodynia.

1.2.1 Neuropathy affecting the sensory nerves can cause the following symptoms

- Paresthesia
- Numbness
- Burning pain
- Hyperalgesia
- Hypersensitivity
- Balance impairments

1.2.2 Neuropathy affecting the motor nerves can cause the following symptoms

- Weakness
- Atrophy
- Gait abnormalities
- Muscle wasting
- Balance impairments

1.2.3 Neuropathy in the autonomic dysfunction can cause the following symptoms

- Hypersensitivity
- Difficulty with manipulation
- Heat intolerance
- Digestive symptoms

- Erectile dysfunction
- Dry skin
- Miscellaneous others

2. Management strategies

The management of peripheral neuropathy aims to alleviate impairments and improve functional status and participation. Pharmacological and non-pharmacological combinations of approaches tailored to individual patient needs are often employed to achieve optimal outcomes (**Figure 4**).

- *Pharmacological*
- *Non-pharmacological*

2.1 Pharmacological

Pharmacotherapy plays a central part in overseeing peripheral neuropathy by providing symptomatic relief and addressing underlying pathophysiological processes. Commonly used analgesics comprise anticonvulsants, serotonin-norepinephrine reuptake inhibitors, and tricyclic antidepressants, which effectively alleviate neuropathic pain. Topical treatments offer localized pain relief, while opioid analgesics are

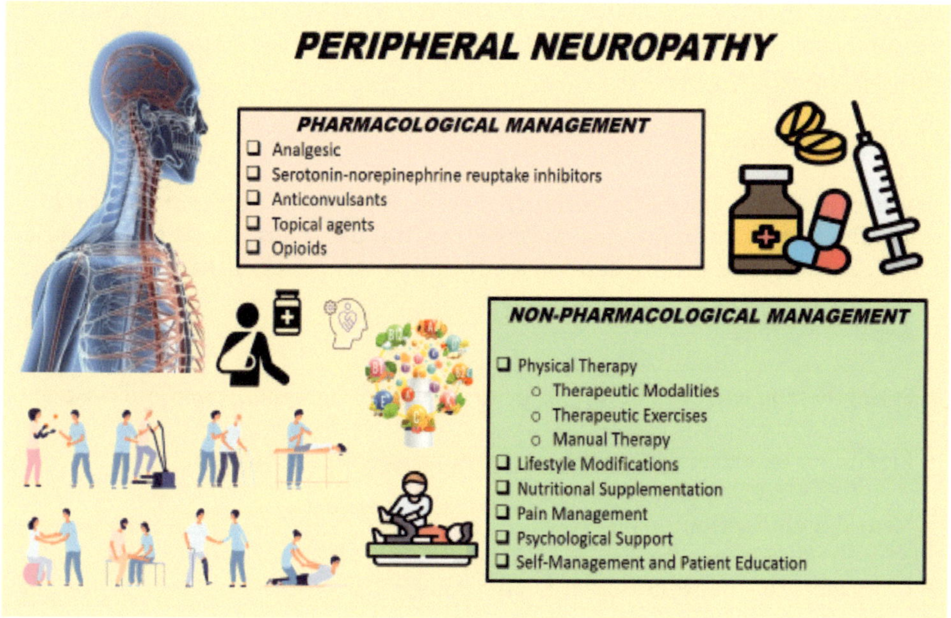

Figure 4.
Pharmacological and non-pharmacological management of peripheral neuropathy.

reserved for severe, refractory cases due to their hazards of reliance, tolerance, and negative consequences [4].

2.2 Non-pharmacological

2.2.1 Physical therapy

Physical therapy is essential for managing peripheral neuropathy because it enhances flexibility, proprioception, strength, balance, and mobility. Therapeutic modalities such as transcutaneous electrical nerve stimulation (TENS) and percutaneous electrical nerve stimulation (PENS) improve pain, reduce inflammation, reduce edema, and improve circulation, tissue healing, and preservation of strength after injury. Therapeutic exercises focus on strengthening weakened muscles, enhancing range of motion, and improving balance and gait. Balance or proprioceptive exercises help reduce the risk of falls and improve functional independence, along with manual therapy.

2.2.1.1 Therapeutic modalities

Therapeutic modalities have potential benefits by addressing impaired microcirculation in peripheral nerves. Its metabolic effects, increasing muscle oxidative capacity, are particularly noteworthy. Its local release of neurotransmitters, such as serotonin, increases mitochondrial adenosine triphosphate (ATP) production, endorphin release, and anti-inflammatory actions. TENS stimulates the underlying nerves and modifies pain perception by applying electrical currents to the skin's surface. According to the gate control theory of pain, TENS has been demonstrated to increase function and lessen discomfort in individuals with peripheral neuropathy. In the context of peripheral neuropathy, other electrical stimulation modalities, such as percutaneous electrical nerve stimulation (PENS), have also been studied and have significantly reduced pain [16].

2.2.1.2 Therapeutic exercises

Numerous studies have been conducted on therapeutic exercises in relation to peripheral neuropathy. Improving glycemic control, peripheral blood flow, muscle strength, balance, and proprioception are the main objectives of these therapies.

- Aerobic exercise.
- Strengthening exercise (isometric, graded weight progression, open and close chain).
- Flexibility exercises (progressive stretching and self-stretches).
- Neural mobilization.
- Proprioceptive neuromuscular facilitation (PNF).
- Sensory desensitization.
- Sensory re-education.

- Balance and Gait training (can improve proprioception and stability).
- Orthoses (ankle foot orthoses).

Aerobic exercise: In patients with peripheral neuropathy, aerobic exercise has been demonstrated to enhance nerve function, lower inflammation, and improve glycemic control. A study conducted by Naimat-Ullah MSW et al. discovered that patients with diabetic neuropathy experience less pain when they engage in aerobic workouts [17]. A 5–10-minute warm-up should be the first part of any exercise program, followed by a 5–10-minute cool-down, which is done by gentle stretching. Aerobic exercise regimens usually include walking, cycling, or treadmill workouts; elliptical trainers, treadmills, cycle ergometers, and recumbent steppers can also be utilized. Aerobic exercise should be done three to five times a week for 30–60 minutes each time, with no more than 2 days between sessions [18].

Strengthening exercises: To overcome disuse atrophy in the early phases of peripheral nerve damage, strength maintenance is crucial. The categories of muscle-strengthening exercises are as follows:

- *Isometric exercise:* contraction of the muscles without joint movement.
- *Isotonic exercise:* joints undergo a range of motion while against continuous resistance.
- *Isokinetic exercise:* similar to isotonic exercise, as it involves movement of the joint maximum resistance is accomplished through managing the exercise's speed.

The American College of Sports Medicine and the American Diabetes Association recommend 2 or 3 days of large-muscle-group resistance training per week with 8–12 repetitions, which includes at least one set of five or more strengthening exercises, followed by 5–10 minutes of warm-up and cool-down with gentle stretching. For example, the wide-grip lateral pull-down, chest press, lying leg curls, leg extension, sit-up, and push-up using dumbbells are examples of strengthening exercises. A study by Kluding PM et al. found that muscle strength, balance, and functional ability were markedly enhanced by a graded resistance exercise regimen [19]. The combination of aerobic and strengthening exercises tailored to the individual needs is beneficial in enhancing functional outcomes [20].

Flexibility exercises: Flexibility exercises play a vital role in correcting restrictions in joint range of motion [5], especially in the shoulder, hip, and ankle. These exercises, commonly referred to as stretching, gentle stretching for 5–10 minutes helps maintain joint flexibility and prepare the body for activities. Stretches that work include toe curls, knee-to-chest stretches, hamstring stretches, calf stretches, and bipedal ankle inversion and eversion. Studies suggest that home-based stretching exercises can lower plantar pressure and increase distal joint mobility in those with diabetic peripheral neuropathy while they walk [21].

Neural mobilization: Many variables, including the nerve's mechanical characteristics, are important in determining regeneration following peripheral nerve damage. Reduced nerve viscoelasticity, intraneural edema, elevated mechanosensitivity, and neural tissue adherence to surrounding interfaces can all be addressed with targeted techniques that deliver graduated mechanical loads to the nerve. However, it is unclear how well these therapies work to promote peripheral nerve regeneration.

Neurodynamic mobilizations appear to be one of these strategies that could be a useful intervention [22]. Neural mobilization techniques for the upper quadrant include the mobility of the median nerve, radial nerve, and ulnar nerve. Neural mobilization techniques for the lower quadrant include the stretching of the sciatic nerve, slump-sitting, and the femoral nerve. According to the study conducted in 2023 by Ali M et al., diabetic neuropathic pain was effectively managed with neurodynamic exercises. Diabetes-related peripheral neuropathy symptoms in the upper limb can be lessened with neurodynamic techniques for peripheral nerves [23].

Proprioceptive neuromuscular facilitation (PNF): It is a method that stimulates the Golgi tendon organs and nerves to restore range of motion, flexibility, and neuromuscular function. Three different PNF stretching methods can be used to target the "target muscle" (TM), also known as the "opposing muscle" (OM), which is the muscle group on the other side.

- *Contract-relax:* At the end of the range, the patient is instructed to contract the TM sub maximally for 3–10 seconds, then relax. After that, the therapist elongates the TM and holds at the end of range for 5–10 seconds, maintaining the stretch until the sensation subsides.

- *Antagonist-contract:* After passively stretching the TM to its limit, the therapist instructs the patient to contract the OM for 3–10 seconds. After the patient relaxes, the therapist extends the TM's range and maintains it there for 5–10 seconds.

- *Contract-relax-antagonist-contract*: The sequential application of techniques 1 and 2.

According to a study conducted in 2016 on patients with diabetic sensorimotor polyneuropathy (DSP), proprioceptive neuromuscular facilitation (PNF) has demonstrated promising effects in treating sensorimotor impairments. The results demonstrate how PNF patterns D1 and D2 are used as a successful intervention to enhance motor and sensory functions by strengthening muscles, reflexes, and sensitivity [24].

Sensory desensitization: Early integration of desensitization techniques into the rehabilitation program is essential for ensuring compliance and active involvement in physical therapy for patients with peripheral neuropathy that causes hypersensitivity or dysesthesia. To reduce sensitivity, desensitization involves gradually exposing the affected extremity to different stimuli. The patient first submerges the sensitive area in a medium, like sand, rice, beans, or Styrofoam balls. As tolerance develops, the treatment moves on to changing the medium and progressively increasing the frequency, force, and duration of stimulation in addition to adding more irritating substances. Rehabilitation results can be further improved by starting sensory re-education as soon as the patient has a sufficient tolerance for limb manipulation [25].

Sensory re-education: The goal of sensory re-education is to retrain the brain to interpret sensory input from residual function following a nerve lesion, especially during the nerve regeneration process. Neural impulse patterns can change as a result of peripheral nerve injury, giving the brain's association cortex sensory impressions that are unfamiliar. By employing strategies including verbalization, visualization, and graded tactile inputs, this method makes use of cortical plasticity to progressively rewire the brain. Basic sensations like pain and temperature are restored first in sensory re-education, which then moves on to touch, vibration, and more difficult discriminative tasks. Using techniques like mirror treatment, the early phase maintains cortical representation of the damaged area while emphasizing the distinction between light and continuous touch. By integrating memory and attention during learning, the late phase progresses to texture discrimination and object identification [26].

Balance and gait training: Due to sensory loss, proprioceptive deficiencies, muscle weakness, and delayed reflexes, peripheral neuropathy affects stride and balance. To lessen these problems, targeted gait and balance training is helpful. These impairments lead to difficulty in static and dynamic balance [18]. Balance training of 20–30 minutes of exercise per session, 3–5 times per week, with 5–10 minutes of warm-up and cool-down sessions, is advised. Exercises on a wobble board, walking on a treadmill, yoga, Pilates, hippotherapy, core stability, Tai Chi, and whole-body vibration all improve gait and balance [27]. The impact of proprioceptive rehabilitation programs on lower limb static and dynamic proprioception in patients with diabetic peripheral neuropathy is demonstrated by a pilot randomized controlled experiment [28]. A 2022 study showed the efficacy of diabetic peripheral neuropathy (DPN) treatment with intraneural facilitation (INF). In patients with DPN, INF therapy enhanced quality of life, gait, balance, sensation, and pain outcome [29].

Orthoses: It is a valuable intervention for managing peripheral neuropathy, offering benefits such as symptom relief, functional support, and pain management by maintaining the affected limb in a neutral position, splints reduce nerve compression, particularly in conditions like carpal tunnel syndrome, and provide immobilization to support healing after acute injuries or surgeries [30]. The objective is to maximize residual motor abilities. Vibrating insoles decreased sway through a suggested mechanism that enhanced early detection of changes in the distribution of pressure beneath the soles, resulting in an earlier response and improved balance control, and flexible polyethylene tubing enhanced stepping responses following disturbances brought on by sensory stimulation from the plantar surface borders of the foot [7].

2.2.1.3 Manual therapies

It has been suggested that massage and joint mobilization may be used to treat peripheral neuropathy by lowering pain and increasing joint range of motion and ultimately enhancing function; these are the goals of these manual therapies.

Massage therapy: It promotes degradation and excretion of the harmful substances by enhancing the metabolism and improving blood oxygen concentration of the tissue so it can improve the nutritional status of the nerve tissue and promote healing. A study conducted by Ferreira et al. demonstrated that the massage therapy program resulted in notable reductions in joint range of motion, discomfort, and functional ability [31].

Joint mobilization: It is a manual technique characterized by small-amplitude passive motion; the ultimate goal is to improve joint play and restore the arthrokinematics of the joint. According to a systematic study by Gordon et al., joint mobilization helped people with peripheral neuropathy feel less pain, have better balance, and increase the strength of their muscles [31].

Physiotherapy plays an important role in treating people with neuropathies. The following is a comprehensive guide about different types of neuropathies, their clinical manifestations, and possible physical therapy treatment options (**Table 1**).

2.2.2 Lifestyle modifications

Lifestyle modifications are integral to peripheral neuropathy management and encompass dietary changes, weight management, smoking cessation, and foot care.

Neuropathies	Nerve involved	Clinical manifestations	Physical therapy treatment options
• Anterior interosseous nerve syndrome	Anterior interosseous nerve	Weakness in thumb and index finger, inability to pinch, pain in the forearm.	Strengthening exercises for grip, splinting, and manual therapy.
• Axillary nerve injury	Axillary nerve	Weakness in shoulder abduction, numbness over the lateral shoulder.	Shoulder strengthening exercises, range of motion exercises, and functional training.
• Brachial plexus injury	Brachial plexus nerves (C5-T1)	Weakness or paralysis of the arm, loss of sensation in the shoulder and arm.	Range of motion exercises, strengthening exercises, and splining.
• Benediction hand	Ulnar nerve	Inability to extend the ring and little fingers when making a fist.	Hand therapy, stretching exercises, and splinting to improve function.
• Carpal tunnel syndrome	Median nerve	Numbness and tingling in the thumb, index, and middle fingers; and weakness in the hand grip of the hand.	Wrist splints, ergonomic adjustments, stretching and strengthening exercises.
• Charcot-Marie-Tooth disease	Peroneal nerve (and others)	Muscle weakness, foot drop, high arches, or flat feet.	Strengthening exercises, balance training, and orthotic devices to support foot position.
• Chronic Inflammatory Demyelinating Polyneuropathy (CIDP)	Multiple peripheral nerves	Progressive weakness and sensory loss in limbs.	Strengthening exercises, balance training, education on energy conservation techniques.
• Cubital tunnel syndrome	Ulnar nerve	Numbness and tingling in the ring and little fingers and weakness in the grip of the hand.	Nerve gliding exercises, elbow splints, and strengthening exercises for hand muscles.
• Cyclist's palsy	Ulnar nerve	Numbness and tingling in the hand, weakness in grip.	Posture correction strategies, stretching exercises for wrist and hand muscles.
• Diabetic neuropathy	Multiple peripheral nerves	Numbness, tingling, pain in hands/feet, loss of coordination.	Foot care education, balance training, and pain management modalities (e.g., TENS).
• Double crush syndrome	Multiple nerves	Symptoms of nerve entrapment at multiple sites; pain or weakness.	Nerve gliding exercises, postural training, and ergonomic adjustments.
• Lumbar radiculopathy	Lumbar spinal nerves	Pain radiating down the leg; numbness or weakness in lower extremities.	Core strengthening exercises, stretching of the lumbar region, education on body mechanics.
• Multifocal motor neuropathy	Multiple motor nerves	Muscle weakness without sensory loss; often asymmetrical.	Strengthening exercises for affected muscles; adaptive techniques for daily activities.
• Nerve entrapment	Varies by specific entrapment	Pain or numbness in the affected area; symptoms depend on the specific nerve.	Stretching exercises for affected nerves; ergonomic adjustments to reduce compression.
• Posterior interosseous nerve syndrome	Posterior interosseous nerve	Weakness in wrist extension; difficulty with finger movements.	Wrist strengthening exercises; manual therapy to improve mobility.

Neuropathies	Nerve involved	Clinical manifestations	Physical therapy treatment options
• Saturday night palsy	Radial nerve	Weakness in wrist extension; numbness in the back of the hand.	Wrist splints; strengthening exercises for wrist extensors.
• Sciatic nerve injury	Sciatic nerve	Pain radiating down the leg; numbness or weakness in lower extremities.	Stretching of sciatic nerve pathways; strengthening core and lower limb muscles.
• Thoracic radiculopathy	Thoracic spinal nerves	Pain radiating around the chest wall; sensory changes along thoracic nerves.	Postural training; stretching exercises for the thoracic spine; and core stability training.
• Ulnar nerve entrapment	Ulnar nerve	Numbness and tingling in the ring and little fingers and weakness in the grip of the hand.	Ulnar nerve gliding exercises; elbow splinting; strengthening exercises for hand muscles.

Table 1.
Neuropathies, clinical manifestations, and physical therapy interventions.

To stop more nerve damage, patients with diabetes mellitus should aim for ideal glycemic control. Quitting smoking is crucial because tobacco use aggravates oxidative stress and vascular insufficiency. In those at greater risk, proper foot care, which includes daily examination, moisturization, and suitable footwear, helps prevent foot ulcers and injuries [4].

2.2.3 Nutritional supplementation

Nutritional supplementation plays a role in addressing metabolic deficiencies and supporting nerve health in peripheral neuropathy. Thiamine (vitamin B1), vitamin B12, and alpha-lipoic acid, an antioxidant with neuroprotective properties, are studied for their potential role in diabetic neuropathy management [4].

2.2.4 Pain management interventions

Pain management interventions for patients with refractory neuropathic pain. Techniques for interventional pain management could be taken into consideration. These consist of epidural steroid injections and nerve blocks, intrathecal drug delivery systems, and spinal cord stimulation. These modalities aim to modulate pain signals at various levels of the nervous system, providing targeted pain relief while minimizing systemic side effects associated with oral medications. Acupuncture, which releases the endorphins that are the neurochemicals that relieve pain, chiropractic manipulation, and mind-body techniques such as yoga and meditation have been explored for their potential benefits in pain reduction and stress management [4].

2.2.5 Psychological support

Psychological support addressing the emotional and psychological impact of peripheral neuropathy, including anxiety, despair, and a lower quality of life, is crucial. Patients can effectively manage chronic pain and improve their emotional well-being with the use of interventions like mindfulness-based stress reduction (MBSR), cognitive behavioral therapy (CBT), and relaxation techniques [4].

2.2.6 Self-management and patient education

Self-management and patient education are essential for enabling people to take an active role in their care and successfully manage peripheral neuropathy. Patient participation and adherence to treatment plans are increased when information about the condition's nature, available treatments, self-care techniques, and preventive actions is made available. Promoting self-monitoring of symptoms, medication adherence, and routine follow-up appointments helps to ensure continuity of care and enables prompt intervention for complications or exacerbations of symptoms [4].

3. Interventional strategies

New treatment modalities and therapeutic options for peripheral neuropathy are being investigated as a result of scientific developments. *Peripheral nerve repair* cannot be completed without undue tension; nerve grafting or tubulization procedures are required. Nerve autografting is currently the gold standard for filling in nerve gaps. However, disadvantages of this approach, such as donor site morbidity and limited length of available graft material, encouraged the search for alternative means of nerve gap reconstruction. Tubulization techniques with natural or artificial conduits are applicable as an alternative for bridging short nerve defects without the morbidities associated with harvesting autologous nerve grafts [32]. *Platelet-rich plasma (PRP)* is a type of bioactive substance that is extracted from autologous blood by centrifugation. A high concentration of platelets can release a variety of growth factors after activation and can promote the proliferation and differentiation of tissue cells, which can speed up the process of tissue regeneration. Because PRP is derived from the body, it can promote tissue regeneration at a lower cost and without causing an immune rejection reaction. It eliminates the neuropathic pain by factors initiating a cascade of wound healing and axonal regeneration [33]. *Nerve Growth Factors (NGFs)* are essential for axonal growth, neuronal survival, and regeneration. Treatment approaches that target NGF signaling pathways are being researched for their potential in the treatment of peripheral neuropathy. In preclinical and early clinical research, recombinant human NGF (rhNGF) and other NGF mimetics have demonstrated promise in enhancing sensory function, lowering neuropathic pain, and encouraging neuron regeneration. In larger clinical trials, more investigation is necessary to clarify the safety and effectiveness of NGF-based treatments [4]. *Gene therapy* helps by modifying disease pathways or fixing underlying genetic mutations; it may be able to treat genetic forms of peripheral neuropathy. Therapeutic gene delivery by viral vectors can improve neuroprotective mechanisms or restore normal gene expression in afflicted tissues. Gene editing tools like CRISPR-Cas9 provide accurate targeting of mutations that cause disease and have the potential to fix the genetic flaws that underlie inherited neuropathies. The goal of ongoing research is to cure different types of peripheral neuropathy by converting gene therapy techniques into clinical applications [34]. *Stem cell therapy* enhances neurodegeneration, promotes tissue repair, and modulates inflammatory responses; it offers a viable treatment option for peripheral neuropathy. In preclinical models of peripheral neuropathy, mesenchymal stem cells (MSCs) generated from bone marrow, adipose tissue, and umbilical cord blood have shown promise as a treatment. MSCs create a regenerative environment that

Pharmacological	Non-pharmacological	Interventional
• Analgesic • Serotonin-norepinephrine reuptake inhibitors • Anticonvulsants • Topical agents • Opioids	• Physical therapy o Therapeutic modalities o Therapeutic exercises o Manual therapy • Lifestyle modifications • Nutritional supplementation • Pain management • Psychological support • Self-management and patient education	• Peripheral nerve repair • Platelet-rich plasma (PRP) • Nerve growth factors • Gene therapy • Stem cell therapy • Neuroprotective agents • Biophysical interventions • Personalized medicine approaches

Table 2.
Pharmacological, non-pharmacological, and interventional strategies.

supports nerve repair by secreting trophic substances that stimulate neuron regeneration and alter immune responses. The safety and effectiveness of stem cell-based treatments for peripheral neuropathy are being studied in clinical trials, and the initial findings are promising [35]. *Neuroprotective agents* target the processes that underlie nerve injury and degeneration to maintain the integrity and function of neurons. In preclinical research, compounds with neurotrophic, anti-inflammatory, and antioxidant qualities have demonstrated promise in reducing the progression of peripheral neuropathy and neuropathic pain [36]. *Biophysical interventions*, including photobiomodulation (PBM), low-level laser therapy (LLLT), and pulsed electromagnetic field therapy (PEMF), provide non-invasive methods for influencing cellular functions and encouraging tissue healing in peripheral neuropathy. These methods work biologically by releasing anti-inflammatory cytokines, improving microcirculation, and increasing cellular ATP production [37]. *Personalized medicine approaches* seek to customize treatment plans based on the unique traits of each patient, such as disease phenotypes, genetic profiles, and biomarker signatures. In peripheral neuropathy management, personalized medicine approaches use proteomic, metabolomic, and genomic data to pinpoint molecular targets and forecast treatment outcomes by maximizing therapeutic results, reducing side effects, and raising patient satisfaction (**Table 2**) [4].

A 2024 study by Gauri Shinde et al. compared treatment approaches for peripheral neuropathy and identified significant differences in various evaluation parameters. Pharmacological interventions showed the highest effectiveness, with an average efficacy of 85%, while non-pharmacological interventions demonstrated symptom relief rates of 70 and 80%, respectively. Healthcare utilization patterns also varied, with non-pharmacological interventions associated with the lowest utilization rates (60%) and followed by pharmacological interventions (65%). Selecting the optimal treatment approach should involve a comprehensive assessment of efficacy, safety, patient preferences, and healthcare resource utilization [4].

4. Conclusion

Sensory, motor, and autonomic dysfunction are the end outcomes of peripheral neuropathy, which is a debilitating condition characterized by damage to the peripheral nerves. This comprehensive review has highlighted the multifactorial nature of peripheral neuropathy, encompassing a broad-spectrum understanding of its etiology, clinical manifestations, and treatment responses. Treatment strategies for peripheral neuropathy include pharmacological interventions and non-pharmacological interventions, in which physical therapy mainly plays an important role in treating patients with different types of neuropathies, according to their clinical manifestations, and new interventional strategies for peripheral neuropathy are being investigated as a result of scientific developments.

Author details

Hafsa Ahsan[1], Wajida Perveen[2]*, Asma Hussain[3] and Sahreen Anwar[4]

1 School of Allied Health Sciences, CMH Lahore Medical College and Institute of Dentistry (NUMS), Lahore, Pakistan

2 School of Allied Health Sciences, CMH Lahore Medical College and IOD (NUMS), Lahore, Pakistan

3 Department of Physiology, Independent Medical College, Faisalabad, Pakistan

4 University Institute of Physical Therapy, University of Lahore, Lahore, Pakistan

*Address all correspondence to: wajida_perveen@cmhlahore.edu.pk

References

[1] Liampas A, Rekatsina M, Vadalouca A, Paladini A, Varrassi G, Zis P. Non-pharmacological management of painful peripheral neuropathies: A systematic review. Advances in Therapy. 2020;**37**:4096-4106

[2] Hanewinckel R, Ikram M, Van Doorn P. Peripheral neuropathies. Handbook of Clinical Neurology. 2016;**138**:263-282

[3] Perveen W, Ahsan H, Shahzad R, Fayyaz S, Zaif A, Paracha MA, et al. Prevalence of peripheral neuropathy, amputation, and quality of life in patients with diabetes mellitus. Scientific Reports. 2024;**14**(1):14430

[4] Shinde G, Mohite RV, Dhulkhed VK. Peripheral neuropathy: A comprehensive review of causes, diagnosis, and treatment. Obstetrics and Gynaecology Forum. 2024;**34**(3s):356-365

[5] Romeyke T, Stummer H. Multimodal approaches in the treatment of chronic peripheral neuropathy—Evidence from Germany. International Journal of Environmental Research and Public Health. 2024;**21**(1):66

[6] Singh S, Dallenga T, Winkler A, Roemer S, Maruschak B, Siebert H, et al. Relationship of acute axonal damage, Wallerian degeneration, and clinical disability in multiple sclerosis. Journal of Neuroinflammation. 2017;**14**:1-15

[7] Hammi C, Yeung B. Neuropathy. In: StatPearls. Treasure Island (FL): StatPearls Publishing; 2023

[8] Laddad M, Bahulekar A, Ghorpade VV, editors. Peripheral neuropathy: A review of epidemiology, pathophysiology, and management options. Obstetrics and Gynaecology Forum; 2024;**34**(3s):635-644

[9] Saylor D, Nakigozi G, Nakasujja N, Robertson K, Gray RH, Wawer MJ, et al. Peripheral neuropathy in HIV-infected and uninfected patients in Rakai, Uganda. Neurology. 2017;**89**(5):485-491

[10] Gwathmey KG, Pearson KT. Diagnosis and management of sensory polyneuropathy. BMJ. 2019;**365**:I1108

[11] Rosalyn E, Septadina IS. Literature review the role of acupuncture in the management of peripheral neuropathy. International Journal of Islamic and Complementary Medicine. 2024;**5**(2):128-135

[12] Shastri A, Al Aiyan A, Kishore U, Farrugia ME. Immune-mediated neuropathies: Pathophysiology and management. International journal of molecular sciences. 2023;**24**(8):7288

[13] Perveen W, Amin I, Hashmi R, Anwar S, Ali MA. Tourniquet palsy in upper limb; a case report. Anaesthesia, Pain and Intensive Care. 2021;**25**(4):535-538

[14] Hanewinckel R, van Oijen M, Ikram MA, van Doorn PA. The epidemiology and risk factors of chronic polyneuropathy. European Journal of Epidemiology. 2016;**31**:5-20

[15] Lehmann HC, Wunderlich G, Fink GR, Sommer C. Diagnosis of peripheral neuropathy. Neurological Research and Practice. 2020;**2**:1-7

[16] Gibson W, Wand BM, O'Connell NE. Transcutaneous electrical nerve stimulation (TENS) for neuropathic pain in adults. Cochrane Database of Systematic Reviews. 2017;**9**(9):CD011976

[17] Naimat-Ullah MSW, Sadiq U, Zafar A, Batool A. The effect of aerobic exercises on pain in patients with diabetic peripheral neuropathy. Pakistan Journal of Medical and Health Sciences. 2022;**16**(04):208

[18] Streckmann F, Balke M, Cavaletti G, Toscanelli A, Bloch W, Décard BF, et al. Exercise and neuropathy: Systematic review with meta-analysis. Sports Medicine. 2022;**52**(5):1043-1065

[19] Kluding PM, Bareiss SK, Hastings M, Marcus RL, Sinacore DR, Mueller MJ. Physical training and activity in people with diabetic peripheral neuropathy: Paradigm shift. Physical Therapy. 2017;**97**(1):31-43

[20] Markvardsen LH, Overgaard K, Heje K, Sindrup SH, Christiansen I, Vissing J, et al. Resistance training and aerobic training improve muscle strength and aerobic capacity in chronic inflammatory demyelinating polyneuropathy. Muscle and Nerve. 2018;**57**(1):70-76

[21] Majeedkutty NA, Jabbar MA, Sreenivasulu S. Physical therapy for diabetic peripheral neuropathy: A narrative review. Disability, CBR and Inclusive Development. 2019;**30**(1):112-125

[22] Santana HS, Fernandes de Oliveira I, Medrado A, Nunes S. Neurodynamic mobilization and peripheral nerve regeneration: A narrative review. International Journal of Neurorehabilitation. 2015;**2**(2):2376-0281.1000163

[23] Ali M, Anwar S, Perveen W, Akhtar M, Hashmi R, Jabeen Z. Effects of neurodynamic exercises on the management of diabetic peripheral neuropathy of the upper limb: A case series. Physiotherapy Quarterly. 2023;**31**(3):53-56

[24] Singh K, Arora L, Arora R. Effect of proprioceptive neuromuscular facilitation (PNF) in improving sensorimotor function in patients with diabetic neuropathy affecting lower limbs. International Journal of Physiotherapy. 2016;**3**(3):332-336

[25] Antonopoulos D, Mavrogenis A, Spyridonos S. The role of sensory re-education of the brain in functional restoration of the hand after median nerve re-attachment. Acta Orthopaedica Et Traumatologica Hellenica. 2020;**71**(3)

[26] Dietz V, Ward NS. Oxford Textbook of Neurorehabilitation. Oxford, England: Oxford University Press; 2020

[27] Køhler E, Dalgas U, Buhl CS, Brincks J. Content and effects of balance training in people with diabetic peripheral neuropathy–a systematic review and meta-analysis. Physiotherapy Theory and Practice. 2024;**40**:1-12

[28] Malwanage KT, Liyanage E, Weerasinghe V, Antonypillai C, Nanayakkara I. A novel proprioceptive rehabilitation program: A pilot randomized controlled trail as an approach to address proprioceptive deficits in patients with diabetic polyneuropathy. PLoS One. 2024;**19**(7):e0305055

[29] Sahba K, Berk L, Bussell M, Lohman E, Zamora F, Gharibvand L. Treating peripheral neuropathy in individuals with type 2 diabetes mellitus with intraneural facilitation: A single blind randomized control trial. Journal of International Medical Research. 2022;**50**(8):03000605221109390

[30] Halac G, Demir S, Yucel H, Niftaliyev E, Kocaman G, Duruyen H, et al. Splinting is effective for night-only symptomatic carpal tunnel syndrome patients. Journal of Physical Therapy Science. 2015;**27**(4):993-996

[31] Al Hulaily ZJ, Al Awad MA, Habeeb TR, Al Haidar FJ. Effectiveness of physiotherapy interventions in alleviating symptoms and complications of diabetic peripheral neuropathy: A review of evidence. Rawal Medical Journal. 2024;**49**(2):442

[32] Carvalho CR, Oliveira JM, Reis RL. Modern trends for peripheral nerve repair and regeneration: Beyond the hollow nerve guidance conduit. Frontiers in bioengineering and biotechnology. 2019;**7**:337

[33] Wang S, Liu X, Wang Y. Evaluation of platelet-rich plasma therapy for peripheral nerve regeneration: A critical review of literature. Frontiers in Bioengineering and Biotechnology. 2022;**10**:808248

[34] Kagiava A, Sargiannidou I, Theophilidis G, Karaiskos C, Richter J, Bashiardes S, et al. Intrathecal gene therapy rescues a model of demyelinating peripheral neuropathy. National Academy of Sciences of the United States of America. 2016;**113**(17):E2421-E24E9

[35] Joshi HP, Jo H-J, Kim Y-H, An S-B, Park C-K, Han I. Stem cell therapy for modulating neuroinflammation in neuropathic pain. International Journal of Molecular Sciences. 2021;**22**(9):4853

[36] Chen Y-F, Wu C-H, Chen L-H, Lee H-W, Lee J-C, Yeh T-K, et al. Discovery of potential neuroprotective agents against paclitaxel-induced peripheral neuropathy. Journal of Medicinal Chemistry. 2022;**65**(6):4767-4782

[37] Zanotti F, Trentini M, Zanolla I, Tiengo E, Mantarro C, Dalla Paola L, et al. Playing with biophysics: How a symphony of different electromagnetic fields acts to reduce the inflammation in diabetic derived cells. International Journal of Molecular Sciences. 2023;**24**(2):1754